Study Guide

Understanding Pharmacology
Essentials for Medication Safety

M. Linda Workman, PhD, RN, FAAN
Linda LaCharity, PhD, RN
Susan C. Kruchko, MS, RN

Study Guide prepared by:

Linda Lea Kerby, BSN, MA, RN-C
Educational Consultant
Mastery Educational Consultants
Leawood, Kansas

Jennifer Ponto, RN, BSN
Instructor
Department of Vocational Nursing
South Plains College
Levelland, Texas

Julie Snyder, MSN, RN-BC
Adjunct Faculty
School of Nursing
Old Dominion University

ELSEVIER
SAUNDERS

ELSEVIER
SAUNDERS

3251 Riverport Lane
Maryland Heights, Missouri 63043

STUDY GUIDE FOR UNDERSTANDING PHARMACOLOGY:
ESSENTIALS FOR MEDICATION SAFETY

ISBN: 978-1-4160-2995-3

Notices

Knowledge and best practice in this field are constantly changing. As new research and experience broaden our understanding, changes in research methods, professional practices, or medical treatment may become necessary.

Practitioners and researchers must always rely on their own experience and knowledge in evaluating and using any information, methods, compounds, or experiments described herein. In using such information or methods they should be mindful of their own safety and the safety of others, including parties for whom they have a professional responsibility.

With respect to any drug or pharmaceutical products identified, readers are advised to check the most current information provided (i) on procedures featured or (ii) by the manufacturer of each product to be administered, to verify the recommended dose or formula, the method and duration of administration, and contraindications. It is the responsibility of practitioners, relying on their own experience and knowledge of their patients, to make diagnoses, to determine dosages and the best treatment for each individual patient, and to take all appropriate safety precautions.

To the fullest extent of the law, neither the Publisher nor the authors, contributors, or editors assume any liability for any injury and/or damage to persons or property as a matter of products liability, negligence or otherwise, or from any use or operation of any methods, products, instructions, or ideas contained in the material herein.

Senior Editor: Lee Henderson
Senior Developmental Editor: Rae L. Robertson
Publishing Services Manager: Lisa Hernandez

Printed in the United States of America
Last digit is the print number: 9 8 7 6

To the Student

This study guide was created to assist you in achieving the objectives of each chapter in *Understanding Pharmacology: Essentials for Medication Safety*, and establishing a solid base of knowledge in pharmacology. Completing the exercises in each chapter in this guide will help to reinforce the material studied in the textbook and learned in class. Such reinforcement also helps students to be successful on licensure exams.

STUDY HINTS FOR ALL STUDENTS

Ask Questions!

There are no stupid questions. If you do not know something or are not sure, you need to find out. Other people may be wondering the same thing but may be too shy to ask. The answer could mean life or death to your patient. That is certainly more important than feeling embarrassed about asking a question.

Chapter Objectives

At the beginning of each chapter in the textbook are objectives that you should have mastered when you finish studying that chapter. Write these objectives in your notebook, leaving a blank space after each. Fill in the answers as you find them while reading the chapter. Review to make sure your answers are correct and complete. Use these answers when you study for tests. This should also be done for separate course objectives that your instructor has listed in your class syllabus.

Key Terms

At the beginning of each chapter in the textbook are key terms that you will encounter as you read the chapter. The key terms are in color the first time they appear significantly in the chapter. Phonetic pronunciations are provided for terms that students might find difficult to pronounce. The terms that were assigned simple phonetic pronunciations were selected because they are either (1) difficult medical, nursing, or scientific terms or (2) other words that may be difficult for students to pronounce. The goal is to help the student reader with limited proficiency in English to develop a greater command of the pronunciation of scientific and nonscientific English terminology. It is hoped that a more general competency in the understanding and use of medical and scientific language may result.

Key Points

Use the Key Points at the end of each chapter in the textbook to help with review for exams.

Reading Hints

When reading each chapter in the textbook, look at the subject headings to learn what each section is about. Read first for the general meaning. Then reread parts you did not understand. It may help to read those parts aloud. Carefully read the information given in each table and study each figure and its caption.

Concepts

While studying, put difficult concepts into your own words to see if you understand them. Check this understanding with another student or the instructor. Write these in your notebook.

Class Notes

When taking lecture notes in class, leave a large margin on the left side of each notebook page and write only on right-hand pages, leaving all left-hand pages blank. Look over your lecture notes soon after each class, while your memory is fresh. Fill in missing words, complete sentences and ideas, and underline key phrases, definitions, and concepts. At the top of each page, write the topic of that page. In the left margin, write the key word for that part of your notes. On the opposite left-hand page, write a summary or outline that combines material from both the textbook and the lecture. These can be your study notes for review.

Study Groups

Form a study group with some other students so you can help one another. Practice speaking and reading aloud. Ask questions about material you are not sure about. Work together to find answers.

References for Improving Study Skills

Good study skills are essential for achieving your goals in nursing. Time management, efficient use of study time, and a consistent approach to studying are all beneficial. There are various study methods for reading a textbook and for taking class notes. Some methods that have proven helpful can be found in *Saunders Student Nurse Planner: A Guide to Success in Nursing School.* This book contains helpful information on test taking and preparing for clinical experiences. It includes an example of a "time map" for planning study time and a blank form that the student can use to formulate a personal time map.

ADDITIONAL STUDY HINTS FOR ENGLISH AS SECOND-LANGUAGE (ESL) STUDENTS

Vocabulary

If you find a nontechnical word you do not know (e.g., *drowsy*), try to guess its meaning from the sentence (e.g., *With electrolyte imbalance, the patient may feel fatigued and drowsy*). If you are not sure of the meaning, or if it seems particularly important, look it up in the dictionary.

Vocabulary Notebook

Keep a small alphabetized notebook or address book in your pocket or purse. Write down new nontechnical words you read or hear along with their meanings and pronunciations. Write each word under its initial letter so you can find it easily, as in a dictionary. For words you do not know or for words that have a different meaning in nursing, write down how they are used and sound. Look up their meanings in a dictionary or ask your instructor or first-language buddy. Then write the different meanings or usages that you have found in your book, including the nursing meaning. Continue to add new words as you discover them. For example:

primary	• of most importance; main: *the primary problem or disease*
	• the first one; elementary: *primary school*
secondary	• of less importance; resulting from another problem or disease: *a secondary symptom*
	• the second one: *secondary school (in the United States, high school)*

First Language Buddy

ESL students should find a first-language buddy – another student who is a native speaker of English and who is willing to answer questions about word meanings, pronunciations, and culture. Maybe your buddy would also like to learn about your language and culture. This could help in his or her learning experience as well.

Drug Actions and Body Responses

LEARNING ACTIVITIES

Terminology Review

Match each definition with its corresponding term. (Use each term only once; not all terms will be used.)

_____ 1. Hormones, enzymes, growth factors, and other chemicals made by the body that change the activity of cells.

_____ 2. Drugs that are man-made (synthetic) or derived from another species; not made by the human body.

_____ 3. The science and study of drugs and their actions on living animals.

_____ 4. Drug action that is intended to kill a cell or an organism.

_____ 5. A substance that blocks the receptor site of a cell, preventing the naturally occurring substance from binding to the receptor.

_____ 6. A substance that activates the receptor site of a cell and mimics the actions of naturally occurring drugs.

_____ 7. The length of time a drug is present in the blood at or above the level needed to produce an effect or response.

_____ 8. Movement of a drug from the outside of the body to the inside through the skin or mucous membranes.

_____ 9. Movement of a drug from the outside of the body to the inside of the body by injection.

_____ 10. Movement of drugs from the outside of the body to the inside using the gastrointestinal tract.

_____ 11. The extent that a drug absorbed into the bloodstream spreads into the three body water compartments.

_____ 12. The inactivation or removal of drugs from the body accomplished by certain body systems.

_____ 13. Movement of a drug from the outside of the body into the bloodstream.

_____ 14. The smallest amount of drug necessary in the blood or target tissue to result in a measurable intended action.

_____ 15. The lowest or minimal blood drug level.

A. Agonist
B. Antagonist
C. Metabolism
D. Elimination
E. Absorption
F. Distribution
G. Extrinsic drugs
H. Intrinsic drugs
I. Peak
J. Trough
K. Minimum effective concentration
L. Duration of action
M. Cytotoxic
N. Enteral route
O. Parenteral route
P. Percutaneous route
Q. Pharmacodynamics
R. Pharmacology

Matching

Match the effect or response with its correct description. (Answers may only be used once.)

_____ 16. After taking an antibiotic, a patient developed an itchy rash.

_____ 17. After taking a sleeping pill, a patient was asleep for 6 hours.

_____ 18. A patient developed pseudomembranous colitis after taking antibiotics for 2 weeks.

_____ 19. A patient felt drowsy after taking an antihistamine.

_____ 20. A 72-year-old patient stayed awake all night after taking a sleeping pill. He reported feeling nervous.

_____ 21. A patient developed hemolytic anemia while taking a drug for malaria.

A. Paradoxical effect
B. Allergic response
C. Side effect
D. Adverse drug effect
E. Idiosyncratic (personal) response
F. Therapeutic effect

Identification: Intrinsic and Extrinsic Drugs

Specify whether each item below is an intrinsic substance (I) or an extrinsic substance (E).

_____ 22. Insulin secreted by the pancreas

_____ 23. An antihypertensive drug

_____ 24. Endorphins secreted by the body

_____ 25. Morphine sulfate given for pain

Identification: Drug Administration Routes

Specify below which drug administration route is described. Then specify whether the route is percutaneous, parenteral, or enteral.

_____ _____ 26. A tablet that is swallowed through the mouth

_____ _____ 27. A patch that is applied to the skin

_____ _____ 28. Injection into the fatty tissue below the skin

_____ _____ 29. Injection into the bloodstream through a vein

_____ _____ 30. Inhaled as a spray through the nose

_____ _____ 31. Injection into a muscle

_____ _____ 32. A liquid that is swallowed through the mouth

_____ _____ 33. An injection into a joint

_____ _____ 34. A cream placed in the lowest 1.5 inches of the rectum

_____ _____ 35. Medication placed under the tongue

Short-Answer

Briefly answer each question below.

36. Who has the authority to write a drug prescription?

37. A patient has severe liver disease. Explain how the liver disease may affect drug metabolism.

38. A patient has severe kidney disease. Explain how the kidney disease may affect drug elimination.

39. After the last dose of a drug is given, a drug is considered eliminated after how many half-lives have passed?

True or False: Age-Related Differences

Specify whether each statement is true or false. If false, rewrite the statement to make it true.

_____ 40. Newborn infants may have a slower rate of metabolism than an adult because the liver's enzyme system is not yet fully active.

_____ 41. Children in the toddler through adolescent ages may have lower drug metabolism rates when compared to adults.

_____ 42. Slower metabolism and elimination of drugs will decrease the half-life of a drug in older adults.

_____ 43. Infants have a greater proportion of total body water than adults.

_____ 44. Reduced kidney function in older adults results in an increase of a drug's half-life.

MEDICATION SAFETY PRACTICE

Identify the correct drug pregnancy category (A, B, C, D, or X) for each description. (Each category will be used only once.)

_____ 1. Drugs in this category have been shown to have an increased risk for birth defects or other problems in the fetus, but the drugs may be given if the benefits of treatment outweigh the risk.

_____ 2. Drugs in this category are not to be given to women who are pregnant.

_____ 3. Drugs in this category do not have an increased risk for birth defects or problems in the fetus.

_____ 4. There have been no adequate studies in pregnant women, but animal studies have shown an increased risk for birth defects or other problems in the fetus.

_____ 5. There have been no adequate studies in pregnant women, but animal studies have not shown an increased risk for birth defects or other problems in the fetus.

6. When reviewing an order for a high-alert drug, what is the best action that the nurse can take before administering it?

PRACTICE QUIZ

____ 1. A patient has been taking an opioid for severe pain for 3 days. This morning he tells the nurse that he is constipated. How does the nurse describe this effect?
A. Intended effect
B. Side effect
C. Adverse effect
D. Paradoxical effect

2. Who is responsible for teaching patients about their drug therapy? *(Select all that apply.)*
____ A. Nurse
____ B. Unit secretary
____ C. Prescriber
____ D. Pharmacist
____ E. Nursing assistant

____ 3. Which of these terms describes the name of a drug that is created by the United States Adopted Name council, is relatively short and simple, and is not capitalized when written?
A. Trade name
B. Proprietary name
C. Generic name
D. Brand name

____ 4. The nurse is reviewing principles of pharmacology in preparation for a class, and is reading about the differences between intrinsic and extrinsic drugs. What is an example of an intrinsic drug?
A. An oral drug taken to lower blood glucose levels
B. Adrenalin secreted by the adrenal gland
C. Intravenous opioids given to reduce pain
D. Inhaled bronchodilators for asthma relief

____ 5. The nurse is administering a drug that will cause the same response as an intrinsic drug when it binds to the receptor of a cell. Which term best describes the action of the drug the nurse is giving?
A. Agonist
B. Antagonist
C. Cytotoxic
D. Paradoxical

____ 6. The nurse is monitoring a patient for an allergic or anaphylactic reaction after the first dose of an antibiotic. Which of these assessment findings may indicate an allergic or anaphylactic reaction? *(Select all that apply.)*
____ A. Skin rash
____ B. Difficulty breathing
____ C. Hives on the skin
____ D. High blood pressure
____ E. Swelling of the mouth or throat
____ F. Bounding pulse

____ 7. A nurse is preparing a dose of medication to be administered sublingually. Which comment best explains the purpose of this route to a patient or family member?
A. "The medication enters into the bloodstream via the gastrointestinal tract."
B. "The medication enters the bloodstream via the tissues under the skin."
C. "The medication moves through muscles into the bloodstream."
D. "The medication moves through oral membranes and into the bloodstream."

____ 8. The nurse is administering an intravenous injection of a pain medication. What is an advantage of the intravenous route?
A. The drug goes straight to the liver for the first-pass effect.
B. The drug enters the bloodstream more quickly than the other routes.
C. The intravenous route is safer than the oral route.
D. Intravenous drugs are less expensive than oral drugs.

____ 9. A patient who has one kidney is receiving morning medications. When assessing the patient for drug effects, the nurse realizes that the patient having only one kidney may result in which problem?
A. Drugs may take a longer time to be eliminated.
B. Drugs may take a shorter time to be eliminated.
C. Drug metabolism may be increased.
D. Drug metabolism may be decreased.

____ 10. A patient has received a 500-mg dose of medication which has a half-life of 8 hours. How much drug is in the patient's bloodstream 16 hours from the time the medication was administered?
A. 250 mg
B. 125 mg
C. 62.5 mg
D. 31.25 mg

____ 11. When administering drugs to infants and children, the nurse remembers which principle of drug therapy?
A. Most medication doses for infants are often higher in proportion than for adult doses.
B. Toddlers, preschool and school-age children, and adolescents usually have lower rates of metabolism than do adults.
C. An infant's kidneys will concentrate more water than an adult's kidneys.
D. Water-soluble drugs are eliminated more rapidly in infants and young children than they are in adults.

____ 12. An older adult is experiencing heart failure. The nurse expects the heart failure to have what effect on the drugs that this patient is taking?
A. The distribution of the drugs will be decreased.
B. The metabolism of the drugs will be increased.
C. The drugs will be absorbed more slowly.
D. The heart failure will not have an effect on the drugs.

____ 13. The nurse is teaching a class about drug therapy and pregnancy. During which stage of the pregnancy is the risk of drug therapy causing birth defects the highest?
A. Weeks 1 and 2 of pregnancy
B. Weeks 3 through 8 of pregnancy
C. Weeks 9 to 20 of pregnancy
D. The last 2 weeks of pregnancy

____ 14. A patient asks the nurse about taking an herbal supplement to prevent colds. What is the nurse's best response?
A. "Herbal supplements are safe, so you should be fine."
B. "Just make sure you take this herbal product at least 2 hours after your morning medications."
C. "Let's discuss this with your prescriber or pharmacist as there could be interactions."
D. "You should never take herbal products with your other medications."

15. The nurse's role in drug therapy includes which of these actions? *(Select all that apply.)*
____ A. Select and order specific drugs.
____ B. Dispense prescribed drugs.
____ C. Administer prescribed drugs to the patient.
____ D. Teach patients about ordered drugs.
____ E. Know the purpose and adverse effects of drugs.

Safely Preparing and Giving Drugs

chapter

2

LEARNING ACTIVITIES

Crossword Puzzle: The Six Rights of Safe Drug Administration

Each clue reflects a problem with one of the six rights of safe drug administration. Complete the puzzle by identifying the "rights" that are described.

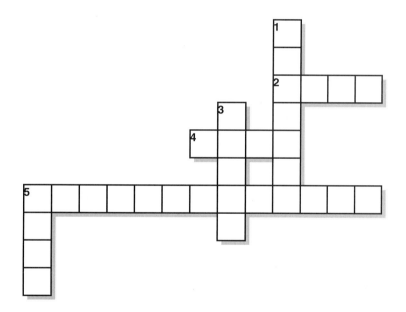

Across

2. The nurse was interrupted during morning medication rounds by an emergency. As a result, doses of morning medications were delayed by 3 hours.
4. The physician gives a verbal order for "IV Lasix, now."
5. At the beginning of a new shift, the nurse sees that a medication that was due 2 hours ago was not signed off on the medication administration record. However, the patient insists that he did receive the medication.

Down

1. During medication rounds, the nurse discovers that the patient is not wearing an identification wristband.
3. The nurse is reviewing orders written by the prescriber. One order states, "Give Tylenol, 650 mg, every 4 hours as needed for pain."
5. The nurse reads the order for "Celebrex" then looks in the drug dispensing cabinet and pulls out "Celexa."

Matching

Match the drug order with the correct drug order type. (Each type will be used only once.)

____ 1. Levothyroxine, 50 mcg, PO daily

____ 2. Valium, 5 mg IV 30 minutes before the procedure

____ 3. Morphine, 2 mg, IV push every 3 hours as needed for pain

____ 4. Give Lasix 40 mg PO immediately

A. STAT
B. Standing
C. Single dose
D. PRN

Before or After?

For each action listed, state whether the action is Before or After giving a drug. (Note: Some actions may be done before AND after.)

_____ 5. Ask the patient about drug allergies.

_____ 6. Check the residual amount of tube feeding remaining in the patient's stomach.

_____ 7. Check the placement of the feeding tube.

_____ 8. Flush the feeding tube with at least 50 mL of water.

_____ 9. Ask the patient to gently blow his or her nose.

_____ 10. Monitor the patient for therapeutic and adverse effects.

_____ 11. Ask the patient to empty her bladder.

_____ 12. Remove the old patch and any trace of previous doses.

_____ 13. Check the patient's identification wristband.

_____ 14. For rectally administered drugs, remind the patient to remain on his or her side for 20 minutes.

_____ 15. Pull the ear lobe up and out for children over age 3 and adults.

_____ 16. Wash your hands.

_____ 17. Measure the liquid drug in a calibrated device.

_____ 18. Document the drugs that were given.

_____ 19. Select an appropriate needle for the injection.

Fill in the Blank

Complete each statement that describes how each type of injection is given.

20. Intradermal drugs are injected _____. The length and gauge of the needle is _____ and the amount injected is _____ to _____ mL. The needle is inserted at a _____-degree angle, and the bevel is facing _____.

21. Subcutaneous drugs are injected _____. The length and gauge of the needle is _____. The needle is inserted at a _____-degree angle for most patients, but a _____-degree angle may be needed for obese patients. Typical amounts for these injections are _____ to _____ mL.

22. Intramuscular drugs are injected _____. Needles for these injections are _____ inches in length, and _____ gauge in size. The needle is inserted at a _____-degree angle for the injection. For an adult, the maximum amount that can be injected is _____ mL; for infants and children the amount is _____ mL.

True or False: Drug Administration

State whether each statement is True or False. If the statement is false, rewrite it to make it true.

_____ 23. Aspirate by pulling back on the plunger of the syringe after injecting a subcutaneous dose of heparin or insulin.

_____ 24. Intradermal drugs are given in the inner part of the forearm.

_____ 25. Remove the needle and discard the needle and syringe, without injecting the drug, if blood is seen in the syringe when aspirating during an intramuscular injection.

_____ 26. Place the sublingual tablet between the cheek and the molar teeth of the upper jaw.

_____ 27. When giving ear drops to a child under the age of 3 years, pull the ear lobe down and back.

_____ 28. Teach the patient not to swallow or chew a sublingual or buccal tablet while it is dissolving in the mouth.

_____ 29. A drug given by the intravenous route is injected directly into a vein.

_____ 30. The Z-track method for intramuscular (IM) injections is used for all IM injections.

_____ 31. After giving medications, reattach the nasogastric tube to suction.

Matching

Match each nursing intervention to its appropriate drug route. (Drug routes may be used more than once, and all options may not be used.)

_____ 32. Inject into the fatty tissues between the skin and the muscle layers.

_____ 33. Use a 1- to 1.5-inch, 20- to 22-gauge needle for the injection.

_____ 34. Be sure the patient can swallow.

_____ 35. Use a 3/8-inch, 25-gauge needle, and 0.01 to 0.1 mL of fluid for the injection.

_____ 36. Remove the old patch and clean the skin thoroughly.

_____ 37. Have the patient lie down for 15 to 20 minutes after receiving the drug.

_____ 38. Use the Z-track technique when injecting drugs that are irritating.

_____ 39. Check the gastric residual before giving the medications.

_____ 40. Place the tablet between the cheek and the molar teeth of the upper jaw.

_____ 41. Stop the medication if fluid collects in the tissues.

_____ 42. Do not give if the patient is experiencing diarrhea.

_____ 43. Give the injection into the space between the epidermis and the dermis layers of the skin.

_____ 44. Potential injection sites include the deltoid, vastus lateralis, and dorsogluteal areas.

_____ 45. Use a 3/8-inch, 25- to 27-gauge needle with 0.5 to 1 mL of fluid for the injection.

_____ 46. Wash hands.

A. Oral
B. Rectal
C. Intradermal
D. Subcutaneous
E. Intramuscular
F. Nasogastric tube
G. Intravenous
H. Buccal
I. Sublingual
J. Nasal
K. Vaginal
L. Topical/Transdermal
M. All routes

MEDICATION SAFETY PRACTICE

For each statement or scenario, identify whether the action is Correct or Incorrect. If incorrect, rewrite the statement to make the action correct.

_____ 1. After giving an injection, the nurse puts the cap back on the needle before placing it into a sharps container.

_____ 2. The nurse enters a patient's room to give morning medications, but the patient is in the bathroom. The patient asks the nurse to leave the medications on the bedside table, which the nurse does.

_____ 3. A nurse draws up an injection into a syringe, then asks another nurse to administer it because a different patient needs to be checked immediately.

_____ 4. The nurse chooses the dorsogluteal injection site for an intramuscular injection for an infant.

_____ 5. The nurse notices that a drug error was made, and reports it immediately.

_____ 6. The patient states, "I can't swallow that capsule." The nurse decides to open the capsule and give the patient the contents.

_____ 7. The nurse is giving medications and stays at the bedside until the drugs are swallowed.

_____ 8. The nurse assists the patient to the left Sims' position before giving a rectal suppository.

_____ 9. The nurse is preparing to give a vaccination to a 16-year-old patient and chooses the deltoid site.

_____ 10. Before giving an intravenous infusion, the nurse removes all the air from the tubing.

_____ 11. The nurse is giving medications, but the patient states, "I don't recognize that pill. Are you sure it is right?" The nurse decides to check the order before giving the medication.

Are Gloves Needed?

For each drug administration route listed below, mark "Y" for "yes" if gloves are needed for administration or "N" for "no" if gloves are not needed.

____ 12. Oral tablet

____ 13. Oral liquid

____ 14. Rectal suppository

____ 15. Intradermal injection

____ 16. Subcutaneous injection

____ 17. Intravenous piggyback drug

____ 18. Sublingual tablet

____ 19. Ear drops

____ 20. Transdermal patch

____ 21. Vaginal cream

PRACTICE QUIZ

1. The nurse is administering medications to a patient who is new to the unit. What will the nurse do to ensure that the right patient is receiving the right drugs? *(Select all that apply.)*
   ____ A. Check the patient's name on the wristband.
   ____ B. Ask the patient to state his or her name and birthdate.
   ____ C. Check the patient's birthdate on the wristband.
   ____ D. Check the patient's identification number.
   ____ E. Check the patient's room number.

____ 2. A patient needs an oral dose of acetaminophen every 4 hours if the patient's oral temperature reaches 101.5° F (38.6° C) or above. The nurse recognizes this as which type of order?
   A. PRN
   B. STAT
   C. Single
   D. Standing

____ 3. The nurse is preparing to administer a drug and performs a dosage calculation. Which is the best action by the nurse to prevent drug errors?
   A. Use a calculator for the dosage calculation.
   B. Perform the calculation twice.
   C. Check the dosage calculation with a coworker.
   D. Look up the dosage in a drug resource book.

____ 4. The nurse is administering morning medications and assesses the patient first. The patient states, "Ever since I started that yellow pill, I've felt dizzy and nauseated." What should the nurse do next?
   A. Assure the patient that this is normal.
   B. Administer the drug.
   C. Wait an hour before giving the drug.
   D. Hold the drug and notify the prescriber.

____ 5. The nurse is preparing to give medications through a nasogastric tube. When testing with an end-tidal CO_2 detector, the nurse notes the presence of CO_2. What should the nurse do next?
   A. Administer the medications.
   B. Flush the tubing with 50 mL of water.
   C. Attach the tubing to suction.
   D. Hold the medications.

____ 6. The nurse is preparing to give an intramuscular injection to an adult patient. Upon checking the dosage, the volume of the injection is 3.2 mL. Which action by the nurse is appropriate?
   A. Give the entire amount in one injection.
   B. Divide the dose and give two injections.
   C. Use the Z-track method to administer the injection.
   D. Hold the injection and notify the prescriber.

____ 7. The nurse is working with a new graduate nurse and preparing to administer a topical cream to a patient's skin. Which action by the graduate nurse reflects a need for further teaching?
   A. Performing handwashing and applying gloves before giving the medication
   B. Cleaning the patient's skin before applying the medication
   C. Shaving the patient's hair off the site before applying the medication
   D. Applying a smooth, thin layer to the patient's skin

____ 8. The nurse is teaching a patient's wife how to administer ear drops to her husband. Which action by the wife indicates a need for further teaching?
   A. Pulling the ear lobe down and back to give the eardrops
   B. Pulling the ear lobe up and out to give the eardrops
   C. Asking her husband to lie on his side for at least 5 minutes after giving the drops
   D. Administering the drug without letting the ear dropper touch the ear

_____ 9. The nurse has just administered morning medications to a patient with hypertension. Which immediate action by the nurse is most appropriate at this time?
   A. Checking the patient's blood pressure
   B. Assessing the patient's pain level
   C. Teaching the patient the purpose of the medication
   D. Documenting the medication given

_____ 10. The nurse is preparing to give a crushed oral medication to a 3-year-old child. Which statement by the nurse is appropriate?
   A. "Here is some candy for you!"
   B. "This medicine tastes really good!"
   C. "Would you like to take it with apple juice or fruit punch?"
   D. "Would you like me to mix this in a glass of orange juice?"

Teaching Patients About Drug Therapy

LEARNING ACTIVITIES

Terminology Review

Match each definition with its corresponding term. (Use each term only once.)

_____ 1. The study and principles of how children learn

_____ 2. The study and principles of how adults learn

_____ 3. The learning area of intellectual ability

_____ 4. The learning area concerned with attitudes, values, interests, and adjustment

_____ 5. The learning area concerned with motor skills

_____ 6. Acquiring new knowledge that results in a persistent change of behavior

_____ 7. The art and science of helping a person learn

A. Affective
B. Cognitive
C. Psychomotor
D. Teaching
E. Learning
F. Pedagogy
G. Andragogy

Matching

For each learning activity listed, identify the appropriate domain of learning. (Domains will be used more than once.)

_____ 8.   Teaching a patient about the side effects of a new drug

_____ 9.   Teaching a patient how to use an inhaler

_____ 10. Explaining to a patient about the importance of keeping a diary of blood glucose results

_____ 11. Teaching a patient how to apply transdermal medication patches

_____ 12. Emphasizing to a patient the need to take all the doses of a 2-week course of antibiotics

_____ 13. Teaching a patient when to take sublingual nitroglycerin tablets

_____ 14. Teaching a patient how to use a prefilled insulin injection syringe

_____ 15. Encouraging a patient to keep a log of blood pressure measurements

_____ 16. Encouraging a patient to teach a younger family member how to administer medication

_____ 17. Teaching a patient about which foods to avoid while taking a specific medication

A. Affective
B. Cognitive
C. Psychomotor

Short Answer: Communication and Cultural Issues

Briefly answer each question below.

18. What is the best way to establish teaching/learning communication between a patient and the nurse?

19. Name three actions to take when *actively listening* to a patient.

20. State five ways to enhance effective communication with a patient during a teaching session.

21. During a teaching session, you discover that the patient does not speak English well, and you cannot speak his native language. What should you do?

22. Name at least four common American gestures that may be considered offensive in other cultures.

Identification: Principles of Adult Learning

For each example below, state which principle of adult learning is illustrated as outlined in Box 3-3, p. 50, in the textbook. (Some examples may use more than one principle.)

23. After teaching a patient how to test his blood glucose level in the morning, the nurse watches the patient perform the test before lunch is served.

24. During a teaching session about diabetes and foot care, the nurse provides each participant with a small mirror to use when examining feet.

25. Before beginning a teaching session about thyroid disease, the nurse asks the patient, "Do you have any questions about the drug therapy?" The patient says, "Yes, I'm worried that I will never get better. How long does it take for the medicine to start helping?" The nurse then answers the patient's question.

26. At the beginning of a class on prevention of osteoporosis, the nurse asks the participants "Tell me what you know about osteoporosis."

27. While watching a patient self-administer eye drops, the nurse notices that the patient instilled one drop in each eye instead of two drops, and that he squeezed his eyelids tightly together after the drop was given. The nurse reviews the dosage and the correct technique for giving eye drops with the patient.

28. After teaching a patient how to use a metered-dose inhaler, the nurse observes the patient's technique each time the inhaler dose is due.

29. During the first session with a patient who will be learning self-administration of insulin injections, the nurse teaches the patient how to draw insulin out of the vial with a syringe. The next session will be about giving the injection to himself.

Short Answer: Teaching Older Adults

List some appropriate tips for teaching the older adult in each scenario.

30. The older adult is hard of hearing in his left ear.

31. The older adult has prescriptions for five medications; some are taken in the morning, some at night, and one of the medications is taken twice a day.

32. The older adult has macular degeneration and therefore cannot see well, but her hearing is normal.

33. The older adult is confused because of Alzheimer's disease, but his wife is at the bedside. You need to provide information about the side effects of his new prescriptions.

MEDICATION SAFETY PRACTICE

State the nurse's best response for teaching in each situation.

1. During an office visit, an older adult patient tells the nurse, "I still have my other pills from the last time I had this pneumonia. I can just take those, right?"

2. The older patient tells the nurse "I have so many pills to take that I can't keep them straight! Now the doctor is giving me two more prescriptions and tells me to take calcium twice a day? What can I do?"

3. A patient calls the office and says, "I forgot to take my blood pressure pill. I'm supposed to take it twice a day. It's almost time for the other one, so can I take both of them now?"

PRACTICE QUIZ

_____ 1. A 72-year-old patient has several new prescriptions and tells the nurse that she is afraid that she will forget to take them. Which action by the nurse would be most helpful in this situation?
   A. Tell her that she will get used to the routine after a few days.
   B. Remind the patient how important it is to take her medications correctly.
   C. Instruct the patient to buy a pill organizer.
   D. Assist her with creating a chart that specifies when each medication is due each day.

_____ 2. The nurse has reviewed a low-salt diet with a patient who has a prescription for high blood pressure medication. This reflects learning in which domain?
   A. Physical
   B. Cognitive
   C. Affective
   D. Psychomotor

_____ 3. The nurse is setting up a teaching session with a 78-year-old patient who will be going home on medications to lower cholesterol levels. Which education strategy best reflects consideration of changes that occur with aging?
   A. Show the patient a video about cholesterol-lowering drugs.
   B. Wait until the patient is discharged before starting the education session.
   C. Give the patient large-print handouts that reflect the verbal information presented during the session.
   D. Give the patient the prescribing information that comes with the medication.

_____ 4. Which action is the first step the nurse should take when planning a teaching session?
   A. Present simple concepts before presenting complex concepts.
   B. Determine what the patient already knows about the topic.
   C. Allow time for practice.
   D. Reinforce learning and provide correction as needed.

_____ 5. During a teaching session, the nurse observes the patient for signs of active participation. Which patient behavior would indicate that the patient needs to take a more active role in his learning?
   A. Asking questions during the session
   B. Taking notes during the session
   C. Checking the clock often during the session
   D. Answering questions when asked

6. The nurse uses principles of andragogy when planning education sessions for adults. Which of these statements reflects andragogy? (_Select all that apply._)
   _____ A. The learner understands why learning is needed for a specific situation.
   _____ B. The learner feels a sense of accomplishment when learning has occurred.
   _____ C. Complex topics are taught at the beginning of teaching sessions.
   _____ D. The learner takes responsibility for learning.
   _____ E. Giving feedback is avoided if the feedback may be upsetting to the patient.

_____ 7. A patient needs to have a teaching session about new oral drug therapy for his type 2 diabetes. The nurse is trying to choose a time that would best enhance communication with the patient. Which situation would be the best choice for this teaching session?
   A. Just after a pain medication has been given
   B. In the morning after the patient has had a bath and is sitting in the chair
   C. In the afternoon just before lunch
   D. Later in the evening after visitors have left for the day

_____ 8. The nurse is discussing a new medication with a patient who is Native American and notices that the patient has remained silent during the conversation. What should the nurse do?

A. Allow time for silence before talking again to the patient.

B. Tell the patient you will return when he or she feels like talking.

C. Ask the patient, "Have I said something to upset you?"

D. Repeat the information in case the patient did not hear correctly.

Medical Systems of Weights and Measures

LEARNING ACTIVITIES

Crossword Puzzle: Terminology Review

Each clue defines a key term in weights and measures. Complete the puzzle by identifying the key terms that are described.

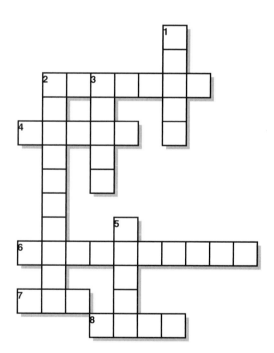

Across
2. One name for the metric system method of measuring temperature
4. Heparin and insulin are measured in _____
6. The system used in the U.S. for measuring temperature
7. The abbreviation of the unit used to measure electrolytes
8. The basic unit of weight used in the metric system

Down
1. Patients most often use this dry household measure to report their weight
2. Another name for the term in 2 across
3. The basic unit of liquid in the metric system
5. The basic unit of length in the metric system

Equivalents

Complete the following equivalents.

1. 1 pound = _____ ounces

2. _____ teaspoons = 1 tablespoon

3. 1 cup = _____ ounces

4. 1 gallon = _____ quarts

5. _____ feet = 1 yard

6. $32°$ F = _____ $°$ C

7. 1 kilogram = _____ grams

8. 1 gram = _____ milligrams

9. 1 liter = _____ milliliters

10. 1 centimeter = _____ millimeters

11. _____ pounds = 1 kilogram

12. 1 teaspoon = _____ milliliter(s)

13. _____ drops = 1 milliliter

14. 15 milliliters = _____ tablespoon(s)

15. 1 fluid ounce = _____ milliliter(s)

Prefixes

For each prefix list the correct unit of measure and its abbreviation.

16. "kilo"   Weight: _____   Length: _____

17. "micro"   Weight: _____

18. "deci"   Liquids: _____

19. "centi"   Length: _____

20. "milli"   Weight: _____   Liquids: _____   Length: _____

21. "nano"   Weight: _____

MEDICATION SAFETY PRACTICE

State whether each statement is True or False. If the statement is false, rewrite it to make it true.

_____ 1.   A liquid ounce is equal to a dry ounce.

_____ 2.   Patients may use teaspoons and tablespoons from tableware to measure liquid drugs.

_____ 3.   When measuring liquid drugs in a medicine cup, fill while holding the cup at eye level.

_____ 4.   A one-milligram tablet of a drug is 1000 times stronger than a one-microgram tablet of that same drug.

_____ 5.   A person's weight in kilograms is approximately double his or her weight in pounds.

_____ 6.   The abbreviation "U" is acceptable for abbreviating "units" when dosing heparin.

_____ 7.   Milliequivalents are used to measure electrolytes.

_____ 8.   Insulin syringes may be interchanged with noninsulin syringes.

_____ 9.   Normal human body temperature in Celsius/centigrade ranges between 36.1° and 37.8° C.

_____ 10. When giving liquid medication with a dropper, place the dropper into the side of the patient's mouth rather than in the middle where it can cause choking if it runs down the throat too quickly.

Conversions

Solve the following conversion problems, dosage problems, and drug calculations.

11. $100° \text{ F} = \underline{\quad} ° \text{ C}$

12. $39.5° \text{ C} = \underline{\quad} ° \text{ F}$

13. A patient is to take 2 tsp of cough syrup every 4 hours as needed for a cough. Convert 2 tsp to mL. _____

14. $600 \text{ mL} = \underline{\quad} \text{ L}$

15. $2.5 \text{ L} = \underline{\quad} \text{ mL}$

16. $223 \text{ lbs} = \underline{\quad} \text{ kg}$

17. $79 \text{ kg} = \underline{\quad} \text{ lbs}$

18. $15 \text{ oz} = \underline{\quad} \text{ g}$

19. A patient is to receive a bolus injection of 8000 units of heparin. The vial of heparin contains 10,000 units/mL. How many milliliters will be drawn up into the syringe? _____ mL

PRACTICE QUIZ

____ 1. Which unit is the basic measure of weight in the metric system?
   A. Dram
   B. Gram
   C. Meter
   D. Liter

2. Which statements about metric measurements are correct? *(Select all that apply.)*
   ____ A. A kilogram is 1000 times heavier than a gram.
   ____ B. A centimeter is 1/10 of a meter.
   ____ C. A milligram is 1000 times smaller than a gram.
   ____ D. A milliliter is 1/1000 of a liter.
   ____ E. A microgram is 1000 times heavier than a milligram.

____ 3. An order for a liquid medication states to give "1 fluid ounce" per dose. The patient has a medication measuring device that is marked in tablespoons only. The nurse tells the patient that the dose of 1 fluid ounce equals how many tablespoons?
   A. ½
   B. 1
   C. 2
   D. 3

4. Which units are appropriate measures for solids? *(Select all that apply.)*
   ____ A. Ounce
   ____ B. Teaspoon
   ____ C. Drop
   ____ D. Gram
   ____ E. Milliliter
   ____ F. Nanogram

____ 5. During an admission assessment, the nurse documents that the patient weighs 109.1 kg. The patient asks the nurse, "What does that mean in pounds?" Which answer is correct?
   A. "You weigh 109.1 pounds."
   B. "You weigh 218 pounds."
   C. "You weigh 240 pounds."
   D. "You weigh 272.8 pounds."

6. A patient reports constipation and the nurse sees an order to give magnesium hydroxide, 1.5 ounces, at bedtime as needed. How many mL will the nurse give to the patient? _____ mL

7. As part of a bowel preparation before a colonoscopy, a patient will need to take fifteen doses of 200 mL of polyethylene glycol electrolyte solution every 10 minutes. After this prep is completed, how many liters of medication will the patient have consumed? _____ L

8. A patient will be receiving an intravenous dose of penicillin G potassium, 500,000 units per dose, every 6 hours. The medication is available in vials of 1 million units/50 mL. How many mL will the nurse draw up in the syringe to prepare an IV piggyback solution that contains 500,000 units of this medication? _____ mL

9. The nurse is preparing to administer a 10 mEq dose of oral potassium chloride liquid medication. The medication comes in unit dose packets of 20 mEq/15 mL. How many mL will the patient receive per dose? _____ mL

____ 10. Digoxin 250 micrograms PO is prescribed. The medication is available in scored tablets of 0.25 mg each. How many tablets should be given to the patient?
   A. ⅒
   B. ¹⁄₂₅
   C. 1
   D. 10

Mathematics Review and Introduction to Dosage Calculation

chapter

5

LEARNING ACTIVITIES

Terminology Review

Match each definition with its corresponding term. (Use each term only once; not all terms will be used.)

_____ 1. Drug delivery into the body by injection just under the top part of the skin

_____ 2. Drug delivery into the body by injection into the muscle

_____ 3. Drug delivery into the body by injection just below the skin into the fat

_____ 4. Drug delivery to the body that does not use the gastrointestinal tract

_____ 5. The bottom number in a fraction

_____ 6. The top number in a fraction that is divided by the bottom number

_____ 7. The answer to a division problem

_____ 8. The expression of how a number is related to 100

_____ 9. The part of a whole number based on a system of units of ten

_____ 10. An equal mathematic relationship between two sets of numbers

A. Enteral
B. Parenteral
C. Subcutaneous
D. Intravenous
E. Intramuscular
F. Intradermal
G. Decimal
H. Numerator
I. Denominator
J. Percent
K. Quotient
L. Proportion

Mathematics Review

11. For the fractions listed below, identify the numerator and denominator, and specify whether the fraction is a proper or improper fraction.

a. $\frac{5}{9}$

b. $\frac{3}{4}$

c. $\frac{11}{6}$

d. $\frac{2}{3}$

12. For the decimal numbers listed below, identify the divisor, the dividend, and the quotient.

    a. $36.5/2$

    b. $11.4/5.9$

    c. $30.3/5$

    d. $52.5/4.6$

13. Change each number below to a fraction.

    a. 9

    b. 552

14. Change each mixed number fraction below to an improper fraction.

    a. $1\frac{3}{4}$

    b. $5\frac{1}{3}$

15. Reduce each fraction to its lowest terms.

    a. $75/100$

    b. $99/126$

    c. $53/72$

    d. $12/288$

16. Calculate the answer to each problem below. If the answer is an improper fraction, convert it to a mixed number fraction.

    a. $2/3 + 5/3$

    b. $1/6 + 2/6 + 3/6 + 5/6$

    c. $2/6 + 3/5 + 1/3$

    d. $6/8 - 4/8$

    e. $4\frac{3}{8} - 12/8$

    f. $7\frac{5}{8} - 2\frac{1}{5}$

    g. $4/8 \times 1/3$

  h. ⅛ × 5 ½

  i. 7 ½ × 4⅕

  j. 4 ÷ ½

  k. ⅞ ÷ ⅓

  l. 7 ¼ ÷ ⅗

17. Calculate the product or quotient of each problem below.

  a. 0.125 × 100

  b. 11.4 × 5.9

  c. ⅕ × 3.8

  d. 550 ÷ 0.2

  e. 1.7 ÷ 1.7

  f. 6.5 ÷ 0.35

18. Change each fraction below to a decimal.

  a. ⁷⁵⁄₁₀₀

  b. ⅓

  c. ⅘

19. Change each decimal below to a fraction.

  a. 0.25

  b. 0.88

  c. 0.46

20. Calculate the given percentages of each number below.

  a. 1% of 100

  b. 55% of 50

  c. 0.5% of 10

21. Express each problem below as a fractional proportion.

    a. If one batch of cookies yields 12 cookies, then 3 batches of cookies yields 36 cookies.

    b. If 1 mL of filgrastim contains 300 mcg, then 2 mL contains 600 mcg.

MEDICATION SAFETY PRACTICE

1. Which decimal numbers are written correctly? What is wrong with the decimal numbers that are written incorrectly?

    a. .125

    b. .1250

    c. 0.125

    d. 0.1250

    e. 1250.0

2. If a dosage calculation results in the dosage being 1.5 scored tablets, how many tablets will you give? Will you round up or down? Explain your answer.

3. A patient is to receive 40 mg of promethazine IM before a procedure to prevent nausea. The medication is available in a vial of 50 mg/mL. How many mL will you draw up in the syringe for this dose? _____ mL

4. A patient is to receive 0.5 mg of alprazolam PO. The medication is available in 1-mg tablets, which are scored. How many tablets will the patient receive? _____ tablet(s)

5. A patient is to receive 25 g of lactulose PO. The medication is a syrup that comes in unit dose packs of 10 g/15 mL. How much lactulose will you measure for the 25-g dose? _____ mL

6. A medication order reads "Give 200 mg of allopurinol PO daily." The medication is available in 100-mg tablets. Use the proportion method to calculate how many tablets the patient should receive. _____ tablet(s)

7. What happens to drug dose calculation if you move the decimal point in error to the right?

8. What happens to a drug dose calculation if you move the decimal point in error to the left?

PRACTICE QUIZ

_____ 1. In the formula $X = 45/90$, which element of the formula represents the numerator?
A. X
B. $/$
C. 45
D. 90

_____ 2. Of the fractions listed below, which represents an improper fraction?
A. ½
B. 1 ¾
C. ⁷⁰⁄₃₅
D. ²⁰⁄₁₀₀

_____ 3. Which fraction correctly represents the whole number 55?
A. ⁵⁵⁄₁
B. ¹⁄₅₅
C. ⁵⁵⁄₁₀₀
D. ⁵·⁵⁄₁

_____ 4. Which fraction correctly represents 6⅞?
A. ¹³⁄₈
B. ¹⁴⁄₇
C. ⁵⁵⁄₈
D. ⁷⁄₁₄

_____ 5. Which fraction is reduced to its lowest terms?
A. ³⁄₉
B. ⁵⁄₁₅
C. ⁶⁄₇₂
D. ¹²⁄₇₅

_____ 6. What is the lowest common denominator for this series of fractions: ⅝, ⅓, ½?
A. 8
B. 16
C. 24
D. 48

_____ 7. Calculate the answer to this problem: ⅝ − ⅗. Reduce the fraction to its lowest terms.

_____ 8. Calculate the answer to this problem: ⁴⁄₁₂ × ¹⁄₁₆. Reduce the fraction to its lowest terms.

_____ 9. Calculate the answer to this problem: ⅔ ÷ ⁵⁄₇. Reduce the fraction to its lowest terms.

_____ 10. In the equation $3.33 ÷ 2.25 = 1.48$, which element is the dividend?
A. 3.33
B. 2.25
C. 1.48
D. =

_____ 11. Calculate the answer to this problem: $11.4 × 12.6$, rounded to the tenth decimal place.

_____ 12. Calculate the answer to this problem: $7.17 ÷ 11.16$, rounded to the tenth decimal place.

_____ 13. Which number expresses the fraction ¾ as a decimal?
A. 0.34
B. 3.4
C. .75
D. 0.75

_____ 14. Which number expresses the decimal 6.3 as a fraction?
A. ²⁄₁
B. ⁶⁄₃
C. 6 ³⁄₁₀
D. ⁶³⁄₁

_____ 15. How much is 15% of 45?
A. 0.675
B. 6.75
C. 67.5
D. 675

16. The medication order reads "Nadolol, 180 mg, PO daily." The scored tablets are 120 mg/tablet. How many tablets will the nurse give for this dose? _____ tablet(s)

17. The medication order reads "Megestrol, 120 mg, PO twice a day." The medication is available in unit-dose containers of 40 mg/mL. How much will the nurse measure for each dose? _____ mL

18. The medication order reads "Furosemide, 80 mg, PO now." The medication is available in scored 40-mg tablets. Using the proportion method, calculate how many tablets the nurse will give for this dose. _____ tablet(s)

Dosage Calculation of Intravenous Solutions and Drugs

chapter **6**

LEARNING ACTIVITIES

Terminology Review

Match each definition with its corresponding term. (Use each term only once; not all terms will be used.)

_____ 1. How long (in minutes or hours) an IV infusion is ordered to run

_____ 2. Number of drops per minute needed to make an IV solution infuse in the prescribed amount of time

_____ 3. Number of drops needed to make 1 mL of IV fluid

_____ 4. Number of mL delivered in 1 hour of an IV infusion

_____ 5. Result of an infusion of IV fluids that occurs at a much faster rate than was ordered, causing harm to the patient

_____ 6. Leakage of irritating IV fluids into tissue surrounding the vein, resulting in tissue damage

_____ 7. Leakage of IV fluids into tissue surrounding the vein, resulting in tissue swelling

_____ 8. IV pump abbreviation for the volume of fluid that has already infused

_____ 9. Computer-based machine that pushes fluid into the vein by slow pressure

_____ 10. Device that uses gravity to control the flow of an IV

A. Controller
B. IV infusion pump
C. Fluid overload
D. Extravasation
E. Infiltration
F. Flow rate
G. Duration
H. Drop factor
I. Drip rate
J. VTBI
K. VI

Identification: IV Tubing Sets

For each tubing drop factor listed below, indicate whether the tubing that should be used is macrodrip or microdrip.

_____ 11. 10 drops/mL

_____ 12. 15 drops/mL

_____ 13. 20 drops/mL

_____ 14. 60 drops/mL

_____ 15. Used most often for children, older patients, and patients who cannot tolerate a fast infusion or a high volume of fluids

_____ 16. Used most often when fast infusion rates or larger quantities of fluids or drugs are needed

Identification: Problems of IV Therapy

Identify which type of IV therapy problem is described in each scenario.

_____ 17. When the nurse checks the patient's IV infusion site, the nurse notices that the tissue surrounding the insertion site is swollen, pale, and cool to the touch.

_____ 18. A nurse started an IV for another nurse who was busy, and hung a 1000 mL bag of normal saline. After 45 minutes, the patient's nurse checks the infusion and finds that the entire bag has infused and that the patient is having difficulty breathing and is displaying bulging neck veins while sitting up.

_____ 19. A patient had been receiving chemotherapy, but 2 days ago there was a problem with the IV infusion. Today the skin and tissue around the former IV site has started to turn red and peel off.

_____ 20. During morning rounds, the nurse checks a patient's IV site and notes that the insertion site is red, warm to the touch, and there is purulent drainage around the site.

_____ 21. After 3 days of IV therapy, the patient calls the nurse to show a red, hard streak that follows the vein path on his forearm above the IV insertion site. The patient reports that the IV has been "burning."

True or False: Life Span Considerations

Decide whether each statement is True or False. If the statement is false, rewrite it to make it true.

_____ 22. Always use microdrip tubing and a volume-controlled IV administration set with an infant or small child.

_____ 23. Always use a controller or infusion pump with an older patient.

_____ 24. Check the IV site and the patient hourly for infiltration and other problems.

_____ 25. If IV infiltration occurs in an infant, slow the infusion and notify the prescriber.

_____ 26. Scalp veins and veins on top of the foot are commonly used for IV therapy in older adults.

_____ 27. Fluid overload is less common in older adults.

_____ 28. Aging causes the older adult's veins to lose elasticity and become fragile.

MEDICATION SAFETY PRACTICE

1. _True or False:_ Any IV fluid that contains potassium must always be infused with a controller or infusion pump.

2. State three actions the nurse can take to prevent tissue damage during an IV infusion.

3. A drug order reads "Infuse 1000 mL of normal saline IV over 12 hours." Calculate the number of milliliters to be infused in 1 hour, based on this order.

4. Using the macrodrip formula, calculate the drip rate for this IV infusion order: "Infuse D_5W 1000 mL over 10 hours." The tubing's drop factor is 10.

5. Calculate the drip rate for this IV infusion order: "Infuse $D_5\frac{1}{2}NS$ at 50 mL/ hour." The tubing's drop factor is 60.

6. Using the macrodrip tubing shortcut, calculate the drops per minute for this IV infusion order using tubing with a drop factor of 15: "Infuse NS at 75 mL/ hour for 24 hours."

PRACTICE QUIZ

_____ 1.   A patient who is receiving a normal saline IV infusion reports that his arm feels
"cold and heavy." The nurse assesses
the IV insertion site and sees that the tissue around the infusion is swollen and
pale, and the area is painful to the touch.
Which infusion problem is reflected by
these assessment findings?
A.   Infection
B.   Infiltration
C.   Phlebitis
D.   Fluid overload

_____ 2.   Which IV tubing set delivers the smallest
drops?
A.   10 drops/mL
B.   15 drops/mL
C.   20 drops/mL
D.   60 drops/mL

3.   Which components are required for an
order for IV fluids? (Select all that apply.)
_____ A.   Type of fluid to be administered
_____ B.   Controller device
_____ C.   Volume to be administered
_____ D.   Duration of fluid administration
_____ E.   Rate of fluid administration

4.   An IV order reads "Infuse 2000 mL of
normal saline over 24 hours." With a tubing set drop factor of 10, what is the drip
rate for this IV infusion? _____ gtts/
min

_____ 5.   A patient reports feeling short of breath.
The nurse notices that the patient's IV bag
is empty, and that the patient's pulse rate
and blood pressure are elevated. The pa-
tient is also coughing. These assessment
findings indicate which problem?
A.   IV site infection
B.   Fluid overload
C.   Electrolyte imbalance
D.   Phlebitis

6.   Using the "15-second" rule, calculate the
drip rate for an IV infusion of 150 mL/
hour. The tubing has a drip factor of 20
_____ gtts/min.

_____ 7.   Which IV drugs or fluids are known to
cause chemical trauma to veins if infiltra-
tion occurs? (Select all that apply.)
_____ A.   Normal saline
_____ B.   Potassium chloride
_____ C.   Anticonvulsant medications
_____ D.   Chemotherapy
_____ E.   Hypotonic fluids
_____ F.   Hypertonic fluids

_____ 8.   A patient is receiving an IV infusion of a
known vesicant. How often should the
nurse check the IV site?
A.   Every hour
B.   Every 2 hours
C.   Every 4 hours
D.   Only when the patient reports pain

_____ 9.   Which statement correctly describes a
method for checking for blood return at
an IV site?
A.   Raise the IV bag or bottle to the level
of the patient's heart and watch for
blood to show in the tubing near the
insertion site.
B.   Lower the IV bag or bottle below the
level of the IV site and look for blood
to show in the tubing near the insertion site.
C.   Have the patient raise his or her arm
and watch for blood return in the IV
tubing.
D.   Clamp the IV tubing for 5 minutes
and watch for blood return in the IV
tubing.

_____ 10.   Which action is appropriate when the
nurse is providing IV therapy to an older
adult?
A.   Check the IV site and the patient's
status every 4 hours.
B.   Use microdrip tubing and a volume-
controlled IV administration set for
the infusion.
C.   Check the patient hourly for signs
and symptoms of fluid overload.
D.   Use a manual gravity drip for the infusion.

11. A patient is to receive amphotericin B, which has been mixed in a 500-mL bag of IV fluid, over 5 hours. What is the flow rate for this infusion? _____ mL/hr

____ 12. A patient with gastroenteritis and dehydration has the following IV order: 1000 mL to infuse IV over 8 hours. Microdrip tubing is available. What is the nurse's best action?
   A. Ask the prescriber to clarify the rate in drops per minute.
   B. Administer the IV fluids at 125 drops per minute.
   C. Ask the prescriber to clarify the type of fluid to be infused.
   D. Administer the IV fluid using a controller device at 125 mL/hour.

Drugs for Pain and
Sleep Problems

chapter

7

LEARNING ACTIVITIES

Crossword Puzzle: Terminology Review

Complete the puzzle by identifying the key terms that are described.

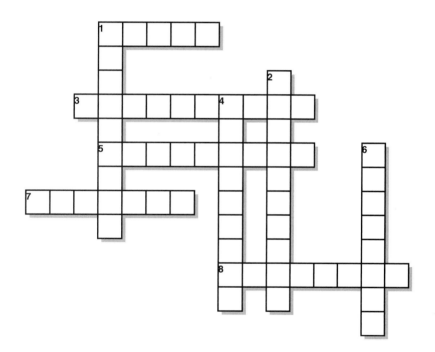

Across

1. Pain that has a sudden onset
3. Autonomic nervous system symptoms occurring when long-term opioid therapy is stopped suddenly after physical dependence is present
5. Occurs when more drug is needed to achieve the same degree of pain relief
7. Pain that has a long duration
8. Inability to go to sleep or to remain asleep throughout the night

Down

1. The psychological need or craving for the "high" feeling that results from using opioids when pain is not present
2. A sleep problem with sudden, uncontrollable urges to sleep
4. A drug that produces pain relief
6. A drug that promotes sleep

Matching

Match the statements about types of pain on the left with the terms on the right. (Not all terms will be used.)

_____ 1. Type of pain a patient feels that is confined to the site where the tissue damage is located.

_____ 2. Type of pain that is sensed in an area that is not close to the tissue causing the pain.

_____ 3. Pain that is felt all around and extending out from the problem causing the pain.

_____ 4. Type of pain that occurs when bones are broken.

_____ 5. Type of pain that may be felt daily for at least 6 months.

A. Chronic
B. Acute
C. Intensity
D. Localized
E. Referred
F. Radiating

Identification: Types of Pain

For each pain characteristic listed, label as "A" for acute pain or "C" for chronic pain.

_____ 6. Often has an identifiable cause

_____ 7. Exact cause may or may not be known

_____ 8. Pain may be described as burning, aching, or throbbing

_____ 9. Pain may be described as sharp, stabbing, or pricking

_____ 10. Improves with time

_____ 11. Does not improve with time, and may even worsen

_____ 12. Unlimited duration

_____ 13. Limited duration

_____ 14. Triggers physiologic responses such as increased heart rate and breathing

_____ 15. Physiologic responses go away over time

MEDICATION SAFETY PRACTICE

For each statement below, label the drug as Schedule I, II, III, or IV, and provide one example of a drug in that schedule.

_____ 1. Accepted for medical use in the U.S., but has a low potential for abuse compared to drugs in other schedules.

_____ 2. A high potential for abuse, but is accepted for use as a treatment in the U.S. However, abuse may lead to severe psychological or physical dependence.

_____ 3. Currently accepted for treatment in the U.S., but the potential for abuse is lower than most of the drugs in other schedules. However, abuse may lead to moderate or low physical dependence or high psychological dependence.

_____ 4.   The lowest potential for abuse, compared to drugs in other schedules, and may be found in cough and antidiarrhea preparations.

_____ 5.   Not accepted for medical use in treatment in the U.S., and has a high potential for abuse.

Briefly answer each question after reading the scenario below.

Mr. B. has been prescribed morphine for postoperative pain control. He calls the nurse to ask for pain medication, and states that his pain rating is at "8." His last dose of pain medication was 6 hours ago.

6.   Before administering the drug, what two assessment parameters are most important for the nurse to assess?

7.   Mr. B. states, "That pain medicine really knocks me out! But it sure helps with the pain." What information is most important to teach the patient at this time?

8.   The medication order reads, "morphine, oral solution (Roxanol), 15 mg every 4 hours, PO, as needed for pain." The medication is available in a unit dose solution of 10 mg/5 mL. How many mL will the nurse administer for the ordered dose?

PRACTICE QUIZ

1. Which factors may reduce a patient's pain tolerance? *(Select all that apply.)*
    _____ A. Fear
    _____ B. Distraction
    _____ C. Lack of sleep
    _____ D. Relaxation
    _____ E. Anxiety

_____ 2. A patient who is experiencing chronic pain would likely experience which symptoms?
    A. Burning, aching, or throbbing pain
    B. Pain felt superficially on the body
    C. Increased heart rate and blood pressure
    D. Sweating and increased respiratory rate

3. The nurse is reviewing the medical history of a patient who will be receiving extra-strength acetaminophen (Tylenol) for pain following hernia surgery. Which conditions may be of concern if found in the patient's history? *(Select all that apply.)*
    _____ A. Liver disease
    _____ B. History of alcoholism
    _____ C. Arthritis
    _____ D. Hypothyroidism
    _____ E. Kidney disease

_____ 4. The nurse is providing teaching for a patient who will be taking a nonsteroidal anti-inflammatory drug (NSAID) for treatment of endocarditis. Which statement by the nurse is appropriate for this teaching session?
    A. "You should expect your stool to turn dark in color."
    B. "Take each dose on a full stomach or with food."
    C. "Take each dose on an empty stomach with a full glass of water."
    D. "Be sure to chew each capsule thoroughly."

_____ 5. The nurse is checking a patient who is receiving an opioid drug through patient-controlled analgesia. Which patient assessment finding, if noted, is of most concern?
    A. A sleeping patient who wakes up when the nurse calls his name
    B. Reports of nausea
    C. Respiratory rate of 8 breaths per minute
    D. Oxygenation saturation of 96% on room air

_____ 6. A patient reports feeling nauseated after taking an oral opioid for pain. Which action by the nurse is most appropriate?
    A. Instruct the patient to take the medication with food.
    B. Tell the patient that the nausea will pass after a few doses.
    C. Ask the prescriber to order the opioid in an intravenous form.
    D. Provide the patient with a low-fiber diet.

_____ 7. A 5-year-old child reports pain after a tonsillectomy, saying "My throat really hurts." The child is to receive opioids. When medicating this patient, which intervention is most appropriate by the nurse?
    A. Use the FLACC scale to determine the child's relative pain intensity.
    B. Recognize that many surgical procedures are not as painful for children as for adults.
    C. Observe for the common side effect of diarrhea, and administer antidiarrheals as needed.
    D. Use an apnea monitor, pulse oximetry, and frequent assessments after medicating the child.

8. The nurse is teaching a patient who has a new prescription for zolpidem (Ambien) for sleep. Which statement by the nurse is most appropriate?
   A. "You need to take this medication at least 1 hour before you go to bed."
   B. "Make sure you go to bed immediately after taking this drug."
   C. "You can take this drug for up to 2 to 4 months if insomnia is still a problem."
   D. "Make sure you have time for at least 3 hours of sleep time before taking this drug."

9. A patient calls the clinic and reports feeling "so tired the next day" after taking a "pill that helps me sleep." After questioning the patient, the nurse discovers that the patient has been taking over-the-counter diphenhydramine (Benadryl) for a week. What is the most likely cause of the patient's report?
   A. The medication is not effective in helping the patient get more sleep.
   B. The patient is taking too much medication.
   C. The patient is experiencing an allergic reaction to the medication.
   D. Daytime drowsiness is an expected adverse effect of this medication.

10. The nurse is preparing to administer a drug for insomnia to a patient who has asked for a "sleeping pill." Which is the most important assessment the nurse should make before administering this medication?
    A. Checking the patient's level of consciousness
    B. Listening to the patient's breath sounds
    C. Counting the patient's pulse rate
    D. Asking the patient whether he or she experiences nightmares

11. A 25-year-old woman will be taking modafinil (Provigil) as part of the treatment for narcolepsy. Which teaching points should the nurse include for this patient? (Select all that apply.)
    A. The medication should be taken 1 hour before bedtime.
    B. The medication should be taken in the morning.
    C. Do not take this medication with grapefruit or grapefruit juice.
    D. Have a family member aware that sleepwalking may occur with this drug.
    E. It is important to use an additional form of birth control to prevent an unplanned pregnancy.
    F. This drug is safe to take during pregnancy.

12. Which interventions are appropriate for the nurse to take after administering an opioid drug to a patient who has sustained a fractured humerus? (Select all that apply.)
    A. If the patient's respiratory rate is 14/min, awaken the patient by calling his or her name.
    B. Warn the patient that pupil dilation is common while taking this category of drugs.
    C. Have naloxone (Narcan) available in the emergency cart in the event a reversal is needed.
    D. Remind the patient to call for help before getting out of bed to ambulate.
    E. Place side rails up and the call light within easy reach of the patient.

____ 13. Which drug is most likely prescribed to treat a patient's pain and burning from diabetic neuropathy?
   A. Acetaminophen (Tylenol)
   B. Pregabalin (Lyrica)
   C. Ibuprofen (Motrin, Advil)
   D. Oxycodone (Percodan)

____ 14. A nursing unit has all of these medications in the narcotics storage unit. Which one has the highest potential for abuse?
   A. Fentanyl
   B. Tylenol No. 4
   C. Lorazepam (Ativan)
   D. Cough syrup with codeine

Anti-Inflammatory Drugs

chapter

8

LEARNING ACTIVITIES

Identification: Infection or Inflammation?

For the following, place an X in the column (A or B) that matches the characteristics of each, Infection and Inflammation.

	A: Infection	B: Inflammation
1. Normal reaction of the body to injury or invasion		
2. Invasion of the body by microorganisms		
3. Allergic reactions (hay fever, asthma)		
4. Non-specific (same tissue response for any location or cause)		
5. Manifests with sprained joints and blisters		
6. Disturbs the normal environment and causes harm		

Multiple Response

7. Which are common side effects or adverse effects of corticosteroids? *(Select all that apply.)*
   ____ A. Sodium and fluid loss
   ____ B. Hypertension
   ____ C. Excessive sleeping
   ____ D. Nervousness
   ____ E. Weight loss
   ____ F. Moon face
   ____ G. Buffalo hump
   ____ H. Fragile skin
   ____ I. Excessive muscle strength
   ____ J. Thickened scalp hair

8. Which are signs and symptoms of acute adrenal insufficiency? *(Select all that apply.)*
   ____ A. Confusion
   ____ B. Muscle weakness
   ____ C. Rapid irregular pulse
   ____ D. Nausea and vomiting
   ____ E. Salt craving
   ____ F. Weight loss

MEDICATION SAFETY PRACTICE

1. All of the NSAIDs except aspirin can reduce blood flow to which organ?
   _____

2. Which is the only NSAID recommended for children? _____

3. Compared to the recommended adult dose of cetirizine (Zyrtec), the common dose for children is _____.

4. A child weighing 35 pounds has an IM injection of methylprednisolone (Solu-Medrol) 30 mg prescribed. Does this fall within the recommended range? Why or why not?

PRACTICE QUIZ

____ 1. A community health educator is discussing aspirin use. Which instruction is most appropriate regarding aspirin use in children?
A. It is frequently used to prevent febrile seizures in children with influenza.
B. It is contraindicated in children due to the risk of developing Reye's syndrome.
C. It is recommended to treat fever and discomfort caused by chickenpox.
D. It is associated with Reye's syndrome, a form of renal failure.

2. Which are common assessment findings for a patient who has used corticosteroids for several months? *(Select all that apply.)*
____ A. Decreased facial hair
____ B. Decreased waist circumference
____ C. Increased fat distribution between shoulders
____ D. Muscle wasting
____ E. Abdominal striae

____ 3. A patient taking corticosteroids should have which instruction included in patient teaching to avoid stomach ulcers?
A. Take the medication just before bedtime.
B. Take the medication by injection.
C. Take the medication on an empty stomach.
D. Take the medication with food.

____ 4. Male patients should be instructed to use antihistamines with caution due to the risk of which side effect?
A. Confusion
B. Hypertension
C. Urinary retention
D. Nausea

____ 5. A patient who is taking an antihistamine that causes drowsiness must be taught that additional drowsiness may result if the medication is combined with which element?
A. Carbohydrate-rich meal
B. Green leafy vegetables
C. Alcoholic beverages
D. Grapefruit juice

____ 6. An older adult patient who is on corticosteroids for severe arthritis is looking forward to a visit from her preschool-aged grandchildren. The priority instructions that should be given to this patient should include information that she is at a higher risk for which condition?
A. Infection
B. Muscle atrophy
C. Weight changes
D. Nausea and vomiting

____ 7. A patient with diabetes is prescribed corticosteroids for asthma. This patient will require additional monitoring for which condition?
A. Abdominal striae
B. Weight loss
C. Increased blood glucose
D. Fluid retention

____ 8. A patient with a sprained ankle asks why the ankle is swollen. On what knowledge is the nurse's response based?
A. Infection is occurring in the injured area.
B. Blood vessel constriction is causing the swelling.
C. Capillaries leak fluid into the tissues.
D. Slowed white blood cell production causes the swelling.

____ 9. A patient taking 50 mg of celecoxib (Celebrex) for arthritis pain should be instructed to immediately report which occurrence to the prescriber?
A. Bruising
B. Gum bleeding
C. Anorexia
D. Chest pain

____ 10. A patient who is taking a COX-1 NSAID is scheduled for surgery in a week. What is the patient at increased risk for?
A. Bleeding
B. Infection
C. Nausea
D. Deep vein thrombosis

_____ 11. The nurse will be administering a daily NSAID to a patient. When is the best time to administer this medication?
A. Between meals
B. Any time
C. With meals or milk
D. At bedtime

_____ 12. A patient taking a leukotriene inhibitor should be monitored for which common side effect?
A. Headache
B. Hives
C. Liver impairment
D. Anaphylaxis

Anti-Infectives: Antibacterial Drugs

chapter

9

LEARNING ACTIVITIES

Identification: Lymphocytes

Identify whether each phrase below describes T-cell lymphocytes (T) or B-cell lympho-cytes (B).

_____ 1.   Keep invading organisms from moving all through the body

_____ 2.   Make antibodies directed against specific organisms

_____ 3.   Trigger antibody production on re-exposure to pathogens

_____ 4.   Work with leukocytes to recognize invading organisms

Matching

Match the terms on the right with the descriptions on the left. (Not all descriptions will be used.)

_____ 5.   Ability of bacteria to invade and spread

_____ 6.   Also known as "blood poisoning"

_____ 7.   Single-celled organisms that have their own DNA

_____ 8.   Drug that kills bacteria directly

_____ 9.   Organism that causes infection when the immune system is suppressed

_____ 10.   Most common cause of death worldwide

_____ 11.   Organism that does not cause infection or systemic disease

_____ 12.   Drug that prevents bacteria from dividing and growing

A.   Nonpathogenic
B.   Bactericidal
C.   Infection
D.   Bacteriostatic
E.   Bacteria
F.   Opportunistic organism
G.   Sepsis
H.   Virulence

Multiple Response

13. What are examples of general surface protection of the body? *(Select all that apply.)*
    _____ A. Bactericidal soaps and lotions
    _____ B. Intact skin
    _____ C. Intact mucous membranes
    _____ D. Body temperature
    _____ E. pH of body secretions
    _____ F. Tears
    _____ G. Saliva
    _____ H. Perspiration
    _____ I. Antibiotic therapy
    _____ J. Normal body flora

MEDICATION SAFETY PRACTICE

1. A child weighing 22 pounds is prescribed amoxicillin/clavulanic acid (Augmentin) for otitis media. What is the correct dosage to administer every 8 hours? _____

2. Penicillin allergies are sometimes associated with cross-allergies to

    _____.

3. A 7-year-old child with a urinary tract infection is prescribed oral trimethoprim/sulfamethoxazole (Bactrim) to take orally. The child weighs 44 pounds. The recommended children's dose based on trimethoprim content is 3-6 mg/kg orally every 12 hours. What is the correct dose for this patient?

    _____

4. List three signs and symptoms of an anaphylactic drug reaction.

PRACTICE QUIZ

____ 1. A patient has been prescribed imipenem/cilastatin (Primaxin). Which is a potential adverse effect of this drug?
A. Unplanned pregnancy
B. Interaction with asthma medication
C. Seizures
D. "Red man" syndrome

____ 2. When administering vancomycin (Vancocin), the nurse should be aware of which serious adverse reaction?
A. Reduced kidney function
B. Impaired liver function
C. Decreased white blood cell production
D. Impaired clotting ability

____ 3. A patient is receiving an IV piggyback containing ticarcillin/clavulanic acid (Timentin) and develops difficulty breathing and swelling of the mouth and throat. What is the first action the nurse should take?
A. Remove the IV access device.
B. Notify the prescriber.
C. Determine the patient's allergies.
D. Stop the infusion of the drug.

4. An older adult is prescribed gentamicin. The nurse will focus assessments on which of the following? (Select all that apply.)
____ A. Intake and output
____ B. Appetite
____ C. Bowel elimination
____ D. Hearing ability
____ E. Joint pain

____ 5. A patient is taking the oral antibiotic cefdinir (Omnicef) to treat a skin wound infection. Which information is crucial for the nurse to include in patient teaching?
A. "This medication may also help your sore throat."
B. "If bloody stools develop, contact your prescriber."
C. "After your skin infection clears, stop taking the medication."
D. "If a vaginal yeast infection occurs, discontinue using this medication."

____ 6. Ciprofloxacin (Cipro) has been prescribed for a patient who is also taking an antacid. How should these medications be administered?
A. Omit the prescribed antacid until the ciprofloxacin is no longer necessary.
B. Administer ciprofloxacin 2 hours before giving the antacid.
C. Administer ciprofloxacin 2 hours after giving the antacid.
D. Omit the ciprofloxacin until antacids are no longer necessary.

____ 7. A patient is taking both a macrolide antibacterial drug and warfarin (Coumadin). The patient should be instructed to observe closely for increased likelihood of which condition?
A. Coronary thrombosis
B. Cardiac dysrhythmias
C. Excessive bleeding
D. Antibiotic resistance

____ 8. An older adult is taking levofloxacin (Levaquin) to treat a urinary tract infection. What is the best action for the nurse to take if this patient develops new onset of pain and inflammation of the Achilles tendon of the heel?
A. Administer prescribed PRN pain medication.
B. Assist the patient in learning crutch walking.
C. Ask the prescriber for a physical therapy consult.
D. Notify the prescriber of an adverse effect.

____ 9. Which patient assessment finding most closely indicates a serious adverse effect of trimethoprim/sulfamethoxazole (Bactrim)?
A. Increased sun sensitivity
B. Polycythemia
C. Skin peeling, sloughing, and blisters
D. Appearance of thrush in the mouth

Anti-Infectives: Antiviral Drugs

chapter
10

LEARNING ACTIVITIES

Identification: HAART

In the following list of drugs, indicate which might be included in an antiretroviral HAART regimen (H), and which would not (NonH).

____ 1. abacavir (Ziagen)

____ 2. acyclovir (Zovirax)

____ 3. amantadine (Symmetrel)

____ 4. didanosine (ddI, Videx)

____ 5. zidovudine (Retrovir)

____ 6. valacyclovir (Valtrex)

____ 7. oseltamivir (Tamiflu)

____ 8. emtricitabine (Emtriva)

____ 9. zanamivir (Relenza)

Matching

Match the correct definition on the right with its term on the left. (Answers will be used only once.)

____ 10. teratogen

____ 11. retrovirus

____ 12. virulence

____ 13. virustatic

____ 14. viral load

____ 15. common virus

____ 16. HIV

____ 17. opportunistic infection

A. Overgrowth of normally present organisms
B. Number of viral particles in a blood sample
C. Virus that can use either DNA or RNA as its genetic material
D. Organism that causes AIDS
E. An agent that can cause birth defects
F. Measure of how well an organism can invade and grow
G. A virus that uses RNA as its genetic material
H. Drug action that prevents viral growth and reproduction

Labeling

In the figure below, label the six common entry sites for viruses.

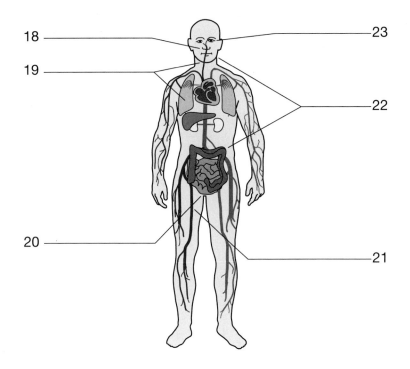

MEDICATION SAFETY PRACTICE

Fill in the Blank

Fill in the blanks with the correct answers.

1. The usual type of tissue through which viruses enter the body are

   _____ _____.

2. Following a regular schedule is critical in antiviral therapy in order to maintain an adequate _____ _____.

3. Before administering ribavarin (Virazole), the patient's _____ and _____ counts must be checked because of the risk for bone marrow suppression.

4. The correct dosage of abacavir (Zaigen) every 12 hours for a child who weighs 44 pounds (20 kg) is _____ mg.

5. Enfuvirtide (Fuzeon) which has not been mixed with water is stored between _____° and _____° F.

6. The risk of rhabdomyolysis in patients taking raltegravir (Isentress) is increased when taken with _____-type drugs.

PRACTICE QUIZ

____ 1. A child weighing 66 pounds is to receive amantadine (Symmetrel) orally to treat influenza A. What is the correct dose to administer every 12 hours?
   A. 2.5 mg
   B. 30 mg
   C. 75 mg
   D. 100 mg

____ 2. Before administering the first dose of val-cyclovir (Valtrex) to a patient, the nurse reviews the chart and notes that the patient is also taking phenytoin (Dilantin) for a seizure disorder. The nurse notifies the prescriber because of which action of the antiviral drug?
   A. Lowering the seizure threshold
   B. Increasing the level of the drug in the blood
   C. Reducing the effectiveness of anticonvulsant drugs
   D. Causing nausea and vomiting

____ 3. A 70-year-old patient is taking rimanta-dine (Flumadine) for treatment of influenza. He calls the nurse at the clinic to report that he has gained 4 pounds over the weekend, and his ankles are swollen. The nurse recommends further evaluation for what condition?
   A. Lymphedema
   B. Pneumonia
   C. Heart failure
   D. Atrial fibrillation

____ 4. Administering ribavirin (Copegus) is contraindicated for any patient with which condition?
   A. Influenza
   B. Pregnancy
   C. Seasonal allergies
   D. Open sores

____ 5. A diabetic patient on antiretroviral drugs has a marked increase in fasting blood glucose. Which intervention does the nurse anticipate from the prescriber?
   A. A decrease in dosage of the antiretroviral drug
   B. An increase in dosage of the antidiabetic drug
   C. Beginning administration of a different antidiabetic drug
   D. A decrease in the patient's carbohydrate intake

____ 6. To assess for liver function in patients who are receiving antiretroviral drugs, what does the nurse do daily?
   A. Monitor the blood urea nitrogen (BUN) level.
   B. Check stool color.
   C. Assess the sclera of the eyes.
   D. Measure intake and output.

____ 7. Which statement shows a patient's understanding of the administration schedule of antiretroviral drugs?
   A. "I take the pills whenever I wake up in the morning."
   B. "If I miss a dose, I don't worry about it."
   C. "I have a printed schedule and I follow it closely every day."
   D. "When I miss a dose, I just double the amount next time."

____ 8. Which intervention will be most useful for a patient with peripheral neuropathy as a side effect of antiretroviral drugs?
   A. Restricting fluid intake
   B. Avoiding apples, prunes, and bran cereal
   C. Inspecting feet daily
   D. Wearing new shoes until broken in

____ 9. A 1-year-old child has been diagnosed as being HIV-positive and has been pre-scribed a non-nucleoside analog reverse transcriptase inhibitor (NNRTI) drug. Which instruction does the nurse plan to include in this patient's care?
    A. Children should not receive NNRTIs until age 16.
    B. Give this medication with an antacid to decrease nausea.
    C. Monitor for anemia by assessing for pallor, fatigue, or cyanosis.
    D. If depression develops, St. John's wort is frequently prescribed.

____ 10. A 27-year-old sexually active woman is taking ribavarin (Copegus, Virazole). Which plan for contraception is appropri-ate for her?
    A. Oral contraception
    B. Condoms
    C. Intrauterine device
    D. Any combination of two methods

11. A patient has been prescribed acyclovir (Zovirax) to treat varicella zoster. The nurse will monitor for which common side effects of acyclovir? *(Select all that ap-ply.)*
    ____ A. Liver failure
    ____ B. Bone marrow suppression
    ____ C. Headache
    ____ D. Dizziness
    ____ E. Nausea

Anti-Infectives: Antitubercular and Antifungal Drugs

chapter 11

LEARNING ACTIVITIES

Matching

Match the possible side effect or adverse effect on the right with the drug listed on the left. (Each option will be used only once.)

_____ 1. isoniazid (INH)

_____ 2. rifampin (Rifadin, Rimactane)

_____ 3. pyrazinamide (PZA)

_____ 4. ethambutol (EMB, Myambutol)

A. Optic neuritis
B. Peripheral neuropathy
C. Reddish-orange stain to secretions
D. Increased uric acid formation

Terminology Review

Match the correct definition on the right with its term on the left. (Answers will be used only once.)

_____ 5. Fungicidal

_____ 6. Secondary tuberculosis

_____ 7. Cavitation

_____ 8. Pneumonitis

_____ 9. Caseation

_____ 10. Induration

_____ 11. Miliary

_____ 12. Glucan

_____ 13. Fungistatic

A. Ability to suppress fungal growth
B. Reddened area less soft than surrounding tissue
C. TB spread throughout the body
D. Cell death and tissue destruction caused by TB
E. Ability to kill fungus
F. "Mortar" between cell walls
G. Inflammation of lung tissue
H. WBCs and scar tissue wall off organism
I. Reactivation of TB

14. For ringworm of the scalp, children may be prescribed the drug
_____.

MEDICATION SAFETY PRACTICE

1. An older adult who is taking an echinocandin is at increased risk for developing deep vein thrombosis. Which interventions can help prevent this? *(Select all that apply.)*

   _____ A. Heparin drip
   _____ B. Venous sequential compression device
   _____ C. Deep tissue massage to legs
   _____ D. Range of motion exercises
   _____ E. Ambulation
   _____ F. Ace bandage wraps to legs
   _____ G. Adequate fluid intake

2. Based on a dosage formula of 4 mg/kg, the correct dose of ketoconazole (Extina, Nizoral) for a child who weighs 22 pounds is _____ mg.

3. The correct maximum daily dose for pyrazinamide (PZA) is _____ mg.

PRACTICE QUIZ

1. High doses of ethambutol (Myambutol) can cause optic neuritis. What visual changes might this include? *(Select all that apply.)*
   ____ A. Double vision
   ____ B. Red-green color blindness
   ____ C. Reduced visual fields
   ____ D. Reduced color vision
   ____ E. Blurred vision
   ____ F. Reduced central vision

____ 2. Before administering rifampin (RIF) the nurse assesses for an allergy to which substance?
   A. Sulfonamides
   B. Aspirin
   C. Sulfites
   D. Penicillin

____ 3. Which statement demonstrates that a patient understands the precautions necessary when taking rifampin (RIF) while on oral contraceptives?
   A. "As long as I don't miss any doses, I will be protected."
   B. "My partner will use condoms until I have finished with the drug."
   C. "I will take two oral contraceptive pills a day instead of just one."
   D. "I will use a second method until one month after I finish taking the rifampin."

____ 4. First-line antitubercular drugs are indicated for which patient?
   A. Pregnant female, to prevent TB infection
   B. Older male taking lipid-lowering medication
   C. Pregnant female with active TB
   D. Nursing mother

5. A patient with coccidioidomycosis has the antifungal drug amphotericin B (Fungizone) prescribed. Which are serious adverse effects of this medication? *(Select all that apply.)*
   ____ A. Reduced kidney function
   ____ B. Hypercalcemia
   ____ C. Bowel obstruction
   ____ D. Widespread skin flushing
   ____ E. Fever and chills

____ 6. Before administering an azole antifungal agent, what does the nurse plan to do?
   A. Administer the medication with grapefruit juice.
   B. Administer the medication with a histamine blocker.
   C. Give the medication at a different time as a proton pump inhibitor.
   D. Premedicate the patient with acetaminophen or ibuprofen.

____ 7. Which patient teaching point is important to include for a patient taking ketoconazole (Nizoral)?
   A. Apply suntan lotion before using tanning beds.
   B. Wear protective clothing when in the sun.
   C. Restrict fluids to decrease the likelihood of kidney impairment.
   D. Apply antiembolism stockings to prevent deep vein thrombosis.

____ 8. A child with tinea capitis has been prescribed terbinafine (Lamisil). The child should have this medication administered in which manner?
   A. To the scalp
   B. To the feet
   C. In the groin area
   D. Orally

Student Name_____ Date_____

Drugs that Affect Urine Output

LEARNING ACTIVITIES

Matching

Match the correct category of drug on the right with the name of the drug on the left.
(Answers will be used more than once.)

____ 1. oxybutynin (Detrol)

____ 2. solifenacin (Vesicare)

____ 3. hydrochlorothiazide (Microzide)

____ 4. dutasteride (Avodart)

____ 5. metolazone (Zaroxolyn)

____ 6. finasteride (Proscar)

____ 7. furosemide (Lasix)

____ 8. tamsulosin (Flomax)

____ 9. darifenacin (Enablex)

____ 10. bemetanide (Bumex)

____ 11. ethacrynic acid (Edecrin)

A. Diuretic
B. Urinary antispasmodic
C. Drug for benign prostatic hypertrophy

Fill in the Blank

Fill in the blanks for each question with the correct answers.

12. A natriuretic diuretic is one that causes excretion of _____ and
     _____ in the urine.

13. The part of the kidney where filtration takes place is the _____.

14. The detrusor muscle squeezes urine from the _____ into the
     _____.

15. Diuretics should be taken in the morning to decrease the incidence of
     _____.

MEDICATION SAFETY PRACTICE

___ 1.   What is the correct daily oral dose (in milligrams) of furosemide (Lasix)
for a child who weighs 20 pounds?
A.   10.18
B.   18.2
C.   20
D.   40

___ 2.   Which beverage should a patient taking bumetanide (Bumex) avoid?
A.   Grapefruit juice
B.   Milk
C.   Wine
D.   Green tea

___ 3.   Which lab test should a patient have done before starting therapy with
tamsulosin (Flomax)?
A.   Hemoglobin A_{1c}
B.   Complete blood count (CBC)
C.   Liver function tests
D.   Blood urea nitrogen (BUN)

PRACTICE QUIZ

____ 1. A patient taking a potassium-sparing diuretic should be monitored for which side effect?
   A. Gynecomastia
   B. Alopecia
   C. Hypertension
   D. Hyperglycemia

____ 2. A patient is being evaluated for treatment with hydrochlorothiazide (Microzide). Which laboratory value warrants notification to the prescriber?
   A. Urine specific gravity of less than 1.0028
   B. Serum white blood cell (WBC) count greater than 4000/mm³
   C. Potassium below 3 mEq/L
   D. Serum creatinine of 1 mg/dL

____ 3. Which question is relevant in evaluating a patient who is taking bumetanide (Bumex) in combination with gentamicin (Garamycin)?
   A. "What is the date today?"
   B. "How many fingers do you see?"
   C. "Can you hear this whisper?"
   D. "Can you touch your index finger to your nose?"

____ 4. Which statements best demonstrate a patient's understanding of treatment with tolterodine (Detrol)? *(Select all that apply.)*
   ____ A. "I need to decrease my fluid intake while I am on this medication."
   ____ B. "My husband is going to drive until I see how this drug will affect me."
   ____ C. "I will change the patch every day."
   ____ D. "I will call the doctor if I get a rash where the patch has been."
   ____ E. "This drug will help stop the sudden need to go that I've been having."

____ 5. A patient is taking 20 mg of metolazone (Zaroxolyn) by mouth daily to reduce edema. Before discharge the patient will be taught which instructions? *(Select all that apply.)*
   ____ A. Slowly change positions from lying to sitting and sitting to standing.
   ____ B. Limit fluid intake to one liter per day.
   ____ C. Increased saliva production can be managed by reducing water intake.
   ____ D. Wear sunscreen and appropriate clothing to avoid sunburn.
   ____ E. Use caution in tasks that require mental activity and muscle strength.

____ 6. What will the nurse tell the patient who is taking hydrochlorothiazide (Microzide) and potassium when nausea develops?
   A. "Hold the potassium until the nausea is over."
   B. "Take the potassium even though you are nauseated to avoid heart problems."
   C. "Decrease the amount of potassium to every other day until you feel better."
   D. "Decrease the amount of diuretic and the amount of potassium by one-half for one day."

____ 7. An older adult is taking furosemide (Lasix). Which special precautions are necessary for this patient? *(Select all that apply.)*
   ____ A. Report new onset of muscle weakness to the prescriber.
   ____ B. Elevated potassium levels may result from this medication.
   ____ C. Instruct the patient to sit on the side of the bed before standing up.
   ____ D. Hearing loss and tinnitus can be associated with the use of furosemide.
   ____ E. Older adults are less sensitive to the effects of furosemide.

____ 8. A patient taking a drug for benign prostatic hypertrophy is having cataract surgery. Which adverse effect could occur
during surgery?
A. The pupil can dilate excessively.
B. The iris can collapse toward the sur-
gical site.
C. The pupil can constrict excessively.
D. The tear ducts can have diminished
functioning.

____ 9. Before taking medication for benign pros-
tatic hypertrophy, it is most crucial for the
patient to undergo assessment for which
condition?
A. Prostate enlargement
B. Gynecomastia
C. Prostate cancer
D. Erectile dysfunction

____ 10. A nurse who is pregnant should not
handle crushed tablets of dutasteride
(Avodart) because of which concern?
A. Dutasteride could induce premature
labor.
B. Dutasteride can cause pregnancy-
induced hypertension.
C. The crushed dutasteride tablets re-
lease a nauseating odor.
D. Dutasteride can cause birth defects in
male fetuses.

Drugs for Hypertension

chapter
13

LEARNING ACTIVITIES

Matching

Match the correct mechanism of action on the right with its drug classification on the left.
(Answers will be used only once.)

____ 1. Diuretic

____ 2. Beta blocker

____ 3. ACE inhibitor

____ 4. Angiotensin II receptor agonist

____ 5. Calcium channel blocker

____ 6. Alpha blocker

____ 7. Alpha-beta blocker

____ 8. Central-acting adrenergic agent

____ 9. Direct vasodilator

A. Combine alpha/beta blocker effects
B. Slow movement of calcium into cells
C. Oppose excitatory effects of norepinephrine at alpha receptors
D. Limit epinephrine activity
E. Stimulate brain alpha receptors
F. Eliminate salt and water from body
G. Cause arterial dilation
H. Block vasoconstrictors
I. Change action of renin/angiotensin/aldosterone system

Fill in the Blank

Fill in the blanks for each question with the correct answers.

10. Diffuse swelling of the face, including the eyes, lips, and tongue, is a characteristic of _____.

11. Beta blockers and alpha blockers affect the _____ receptors.

12. Hardening of the arterial walls is characteristic of _____.

13. Orthostatic hypotension manifests within 3 minutes of when a patient _____.

14. Secondary hypertension is related to specific _____ and _____.

MEDICATION SAFETY PRACTICE

____ 1.   A patient has forgotten to take a dose of prescribed medication for hypertension. What do you advise the patient to do?
   A.   Take double the amount when it is time for the next dose.
   B.   If the next dose is in less than 4 hours, just skip the dose that was missed.
   C.   Since the next dose is due in 2 hours, take the missed dose right away.
   D.   Take the missed dose immediately, and then skip the next scheduled dose.

____ 2.   As a result of reduced fluid volume and relaxation of arteries, most patients taking diuretics are at risk for which side effect?
   A.   Dehydration
   B.   Dizziness
   C.   Dementia
   D.   Demineralization

____ 3.   Stopping therapy with beta blockers should be done on what schedule?
   A.   Daily
   B.   Weekly
   C.   Gradually
   D.   Immediately

____ 4.   Captopril (Capoten) 25 mg PO is prescribed. The pharmacy sends scored tablets of 12.5 mg. How many tablets should be administered?
   A.   ½
   B.   2
   C.   2½
   D.   4

____ 5.   What is your priority action for a patient who develops angioedema while taking angiotensin-converting enzyme (ACE) inhibitors?
   A.   Hold the next dose of medication to see if the condition improves.
   B.   Discontinue the medication and call the prescriber.
   C.   Administer the medication slowly and observe the patient's reaction.
   D.   Decrease the dose by one-half to see if the condition improves.

PRACTICE QUIZ

_____ 1. A patient is taking a calcium channel blocker. Which best describes how this medication lowers blood pressure?
   A. It increases the movement of calcium into the cells of the heart and blood vessels.
   B. It relaxes the body's blood vessels.
   C. It decreases the supply of oxygen-rich blood to the heart.
   D. It limits the activity of epinephrine on the heart and blood vessels.

_____ 2. A patient has been taking captopril (Capoten) for several weeks when severe swelling of the lips and difficulty breathing develop. The nurse recognizes this as which adverse effect?
   A. Neutropenia
   B. Photosensitivity
   C. Reactive airway disease
   D. Angioedema

_____ 3. After administering losartan (Cozaar), the nurse monitors the patient for which condition?
   A. Potassium level higher than 5.5 mEq/L
   B. Potassium level of 4.0 mEq/L
   C. Decreased bowel sounds and constipation
   D. Weight loss and increased urine output

_____ 4. Which statement by a patient best indicates a correct understanding of the nurse's instructions about taking angiotensin-converting enzyme (ACE) inhibitors?
   A. "I'll use a salt substitute to flavor my food."
   B. "After several months I won't need to worry about facial swelling."
   C. "I'll need to use sunscreen and protective clothing for my trip to the beach."
   D. "If I drink alcohol, my blood pressure would likely increase."

_____ 5. Which statement about angiotensin-converting enzyme (ACE) inhibitors and pregnant women is true?
   A. After delivery, ACE inhibitors can be used by a breastfeeding woman.
   B. ACE inhibitors can cause liver disorders in the infant.
   C. ACE inhibitors are category D drugs and can cause birth defects.
   D. ACE inhibitors can cause the infant to develop hypokalemia.

6. A patient who is taking atenolol (Tenormin), a beta blocker, should be monitored for which side effects? _(Select all that apply.)_
   _____ A. Tachycardia
   _____ B. Difficulty breathing
   _____ C. Fever or sore throat
   _____ D. Dizziness when standing up
   _____ E. Hyperkalemia

_____ 7. A patient who has been taking a calcium channel blocker should be monitored for which symptoms of Stevens-Johnson syndrome?
   A. Hypothermia
   B. Gingival hyperplasia
   C. Gynecomastia
   D. Skin lesions

8. Male patients who are taking which antihypertensive drug should be instructed not to take drugs for erectile dysfunction? _(Select all that apply.)_
   _____ A. Beta blockers
   _____ B. Alpha-beta blockers
   _____ C. Alpha blockers
   _____ D. Calcium channel blockers
   _____ E. DHT blockers

_____ 9. Which drug has been safely used to treat pregnancy-induced hypertension?
   A. Valsartan (Cozaar)
   B. Captopril (Capoten)
   C. Methyldopa (Aldomet)
   D. Atenolol (Tenormin)

Drugs for Heart Failure

chapter
14

LEARNING ACTIVITIES

Fill in the Blank

Fill in the blanks with the correct answers.

1. For a headache related to initial treatment with nitroglycerin, the patient should take _____.

2. Heart failure is characterized by a dilated or overstretched

    _____.

3. Decreased renal blood flow related to heart failure is compensated by activation of the _____.

4. Most heart failure begins in the _____.

5. Digoxin increases the force of _____.

Matching

Match the vasodilator on the left with the correct intended response on the right. (Not all options will be used, and some will be used more than once.)

____ 6. hydralazine (Apresoline)

____ 7. nitroglycerin

____ 8. isosorbide (Isordil)

A. Decreased heart workload
B. Increased blood pressure
C. Increased blood flow to coronary arteries
D. Vasoconstriction of arteries
E. Increased venous vasodilation
F. Decreased blood pressure
G. Increased arterial vasodilation
H. Decreased blood flow to coronary arteries

MEDICATION SAFETY PRACTICE

Determine whether each statement is True or False. If the statement is false, rewrite it to make it true.

_____ 1.   Previous doses of nitroglycerin ointment should be vigorously rubbed off before administering a new dose.

_____ 2.   Nitroglycerin ointment should be kept on the patient's skin around the clock in order to maintain a therapeutic blood level.

_____ 3.   Digoxin (Lanoxin) toxicity may be characterized by bradycardia, loss of appetite, and yellow halos appearing around objects.

_____ 4.   The trade name for the drug dopamine is Dobutamine.

PRACTICE QUIZ

_____ 1. A patient taking hydralazine (Apresoline) for heart failure has a temperature of 104° F. His white blood cell (WBC) count has dropped from 8000/mm³ to 4000/mm³. What does the nurse recognize the patient is at risk for experiencing?
   A. Bleeding
   B. Seizure
   C. Infection
   D. Falling

_____ 2. A patient on digoxin (Lanoxin) reports feeling tired and nauseated. What is the priority assessment the nurse makes?
   A. Temperature
   B. Urine output
   C. Apical pulse
   D. Mental status

_____ 3. Before administering nitroglycerin ointment to a patient, what precaution does the nurse take?
   A. Putting on a facemask
   B. Handwashing with bactericidal solution
   C. Putting on a gown
   D. Putting on gloves

_____ 4. Which instruction does the nurse give the patient regarding storage of oral nitroglycerin?
   A. "Keep it in the refrigerator."
   B. "Store the amber bottle in a dark place."
   C. "Keep a drink of water close by so you can swallow the pills quickly in an emergency."
   D. "If you do not feel a tingling sensation, the drug is no longer potent."

_____ 5. Female patients of childbearing age who are or may become pregnant should be told what about taking digoxin (Lanoxin)?
   A. "Drink plenty of water before breast-feeding."
   B. "Digoxin passes from the mother to the fetus."
   C. "This drug is perfectly safe for your baby."
   D. "Try to exercise regularly to reduce the drug's effect on the fetus."

_____ 6. Hydralazine (Apresoline) dosage in children is based on what measurement?
   A. Height
   B. Age
   C. Heart rate
   D. Weight

_____ 7. What is the correct initial dose of nesiritide (Natrecor) for an adult in heart failure who weighs 68 kg?
   A. 10 mg
   B. 130 mg
   C. 130 mcg
   D. 100 mg

_____ 8. After beginning therapy with IV potassium for heart failure, a patient's cardiac monitor shows an irregular heart rate of 60 beats per minute. The patient reports feeling weak and confused. The nurse notifies the prescriber if the patient's serum potassium is in what range (expressed in mmol/L)?
   A. 3.5-5.0
   B. 1.5-3.0
   C. 0.5-1.5
   D. 5.2-6.8

_____ 9. Which instruction should the nurse include when teaching a patient about the use of digoxin (Lanoxin)?
   A. "If this medication causes an upset stomach, take it with an antacid."
   B. "Take your pulse monthly and notify your prescriber if your pulse is less than 60."
   C. "Digoxin toxicity is less likely to occur if you are also taking diuretics."
   D. "Keep all laboratory appointments for drug level testing."

Antidysrhythmic Drugs

chapter

15

LEARNING ACTIVITIES

Matching

Match the drug on the left with its correct drug category on the right. (Answers will be used more than once.)

____ 1.   lidocaine (Xylocaine)

____ 2.   esmolol (Brevibloc)

____ 3.   tocainide (Tonocard)

____ 4.   propranolol (Inderal)

____ 5.   amiodarone (Cordarone)

____ 6.   diltiazem (Cardizem)

____ 7.   verapamil (Calan)

A. Beta blocker
B. Potassium channel blocker
C. Calcium channel blocker
D. Class 1b sodium channel blocker

Fill in the Blank

Fill in the blanks with the correct answers.

8.   The ability of the cardiac muscle cells to fire on their own is known as

_____.

9.   Before administering atropine (Atropine Sulfate), the nurse must assess for a history of _____.

10. To treat digoxin toxicity, a drug is given to bind with the medication and prevent its action. The generic and trade names of this drug are _____ and _____.

MEDICATION SAFETY PRACTICE

1.   Patients should be taught that taking _____ within 2 hours of taking digoxin (Lanoxin) can interfere with the medication's absorption.

2.   Patients with diabetes who are taking beta blockers must be carefully monitored because of the drug's risk for masking signs of _____.

3. To assess the patient's heart rate before administering digoxin (Lanoxin), the nurse counts for _____ seconds. The dose is held if the heart rate is below _____ beats per minute.

4. Children taking beta blockers may experience worsened _____.

5. The nurse instructs the patient who is taking amiodarone (Cordarone) to have eye examinations every 6 to 12 months to assess for _____ _____.

PRACTICE QUIZ

____ 1. Before beginning treatment with atropine (Atropine Sulfate) for bradycardia, the nurse must assess for a history of which disorder in the patient?
A. Multiple sclerosis
B. Muscular dystrophy
C. Glaucoma
D. Diabetes

____ 2. What is the correct dose in milligrams of quinidine (Quinidine Sulfate) for a 3-year-old child who weighs 22 pounds?
A. 16
B. 25
C. 37
D. 60

____ 3. A patient taking digoxin (Lanoxin) reports a weight gain of 7 pounds in the last week. The nurse assesses the patient for the possibility of which condition?
A. Pregnancy
B. Clinical depression
C. Bowel obstruction
D. Heart failure

____ 4. In an emergency, lidocaine (Xylocaine) may be given intravenously or by airway inhalation. Why are these routes of administration used?
A. They avoid interaction with other drugs.
B. They reduce the risk of adverse effects.
C. When given orally, the liver renders the drug ineffective.
D. They are closer to the tissue where drug action is needed most.

____ 5. Patients who are taking tocainide (Tonocard) may have increased risk of infection because of what adverse effect?
A. Pneumonitis
B. Confusion
C. Neutropenia
D. Hypotension

6. Which drugs are used to treat ventricular dysrhythmias? *(Select all that apply.)*
____ A. Atropine (Atropine Sulfate)
____ B. Lidocaine (Xylocaine)
____ C. Digoxin (Lanoxin)
____ D. Flecainide (Tambocor)
____ E. Digoxin immune fab (DigiFab)
____ F. Propranolol (Inderal)
____ G. Esmolol (Brevibloc)

7. Which drugs can interfere with the results of medical tests or allergy shots? *(Select all that apply.)*
____ A. Digoxin (Lanoxin)
____ B. Propranolol (Inderal)
____ C. Flecainide (Tambocor)
____ D. Acebutolol (Sectral)
____ E. Esmolol (Brevibloc)

8. What is the correct dose in milligrams of ibutilide (Corvert) for an adult patient who weighs 140 pounds? (The recommended adult dose for a patient less than 60 kg is 0.01 mg/kg over 1 minute; 1 mg for a patient over 60 kg.) _____ mg

9. An older adult has been given a dose of lidocaine (Xylocaine). Which interventions are important to include? *(Select all that apply.)*
____ A. Instruct the patient to change positions slowly.
____ B. Advise the patient to use handrails to reduce the risk for falls.
____ C. Advise the patient to report episodes of diarrhea.
____ D. Monitor laboratory results for increased white blood cells.
____ E. Observe the patient for episodes of confusion.

Drugs for High Blood Lipids

LEARNING ACTIVITIES

Crossword Puzzle: Lipid-Lowering Drugs

Complete the puzzle by identifying the correct terms that are described.

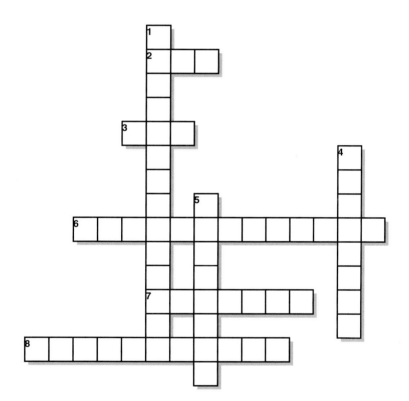

Across
2. "Good" cholesterol in the body (abbreviation)
3. "Bad" cholesterol in the body (abbreviation)
6. Vitamin B that helps decrease cholesterol levels (2 words)
7. Drugs that inhibit production of cholesterol
8. Waxy, fatty material in cell walls

Down
1. Muscle cell breakdown
4. Genetic hyperlipidemia
5. Drugs that lower triglycerides

Fill in the Blank

Fill in the blanks with the correct answers.

1. The side effect of flushing or hot flashes when taking nicotinic acid (Niacor) can be reduced by taking the drug with _____ or with _____.

2. Patients with diabetes must be taught that nicotinic acid (Niacor) can have the effect of _____ blood glucose levels.

MEDICATION SAFETY PRACTICE

1. Before beginning therapy with lipid-lowering drugs, the patient must have baseline testing done for _____ function and _____.

2. Statins should not be given to patients who drink more than _____ alcoholic beverages a day.

3. Fibrates can increase the effectiveness of warfarin (Coumadin) and cause a prolonged _____ time.

4. Gemfibrozil (Lopid) may interact with statin drugs by interfering with their _____.

PRACTICE QUIZ

1. What lifestyle changes does the nurse discuss with a patient who is beginning drug therapy for treatment of hyperlipidemia and hypercholesterolemia? *(Select all that apply.)*
   ____ A. Weight control
   ____ B. Ergonomic work station
   ____ C. Regular exercise
   ____ D. Driving at night
   ____ E. Low-fat diet
   ____ F. Organic diet

2. Although generally safe for older adults, which conditions are contraindications for medication therapy with statins? *(Select all that apply.)*
   ____ A. Diabetes mellitus
   ____ B. Glaucoma
   ____ C. Liver disease
   ____ D. Hypertension
   ____ E. Myopathy
   ____ F. Alzheimer's disease

____ 3. The nurse instructs the patient to take the tablet form of bile acid sequestrants with at least how many ounces of water?
   A. 2-4
   B. 6-9
   C. 10-12
   D. 12-16

____ 4. What beverage interferes with the metabolism of fibrates and makes them less effective?
   A. Coffee
   B. Milk
   C. Grapefruit juice
   D. Pomegranate juice

5. A patient has been taking nicotinic acid (Niacor) for several months and is now at a dosage of 1 g twice per day. The medication is available in 500-mg tablets. How many tablets per day will the patient take? _____ tablet(s)

____ 6. Which intervention can reduce the flushing or hot flashes associated with nicotinic acid?
   A. Give the drug with estrogen hormone replacement.
   B. Administer the drug with acetaminophen (Tylenol).
   C. Give the drug with large amounts of fluid.
   D. Give the drug during or after a full meal.

____ 7. A patient who is taking a statin agent should be monitored for which serious adverse effect?
   A. Decreased liver function
   B. Decreased platelet counts
   C. Increased white blood cell counts
   D. Hypotension and tachycardia

____ 8. A patient asks how statin drugs work in the body. What is the nurse's best response?
   A. "They bind with cholesterol in the intestine."
   B. "They work by controlling the rate of cholesterol produced by the liver."
   C. "They reduce the amount of cholesterol absorbed by the body."
   D. "They are a type of vitamin B that increases HDL cholesterol."

____ 9. An older adult taking a statin agent reports suddenly developing muscle aches and weakness. What is the most important question for the nurse to ask this patient?
   A. "Have you taken any over-the-counter NSAIDs?"
   B. "Have you noticed any numbness or tingling sensations in your extremities?"
   C. "Have you noticed a brownish color to your urine?"
   D. "Have you noticed any facial flushing or 'hot flashes'?"

Drugs that Affect Blood Clotting

chapter

17

LEARNING ACTIVITIES

Crossword Puzzle: Terminology Review

Complete the puzzle by identifying the correct terms that are described.

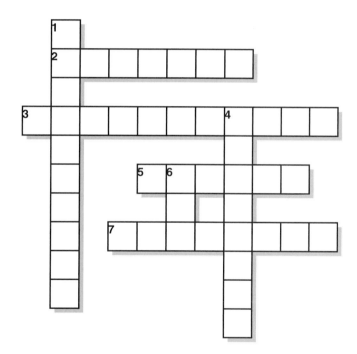

Across

2. Travels through the bloodstream and blocks vessels
3. Process by which blood clots form
5. Protein essence of a blood clot
7. Blood clot in a vessel or within the heart

Down

1. Profuse bleeding
4. Converts fibrinogen to fibrin
6. Blood test used to report results of warfarin anticoagulation (abbreviation)

Matching

Match the type of anticoagulant drug on the right with the correct medication names on the left. (Answers will be used more than once.)

_____ 1.   darbepoetin alfa (Aranesp)
_____ 2.   warfarin (Coumadin)
_____ 3.   ticlopidine (Ticlid)
_____ 4.   t-PA (Activase)
_____ 5.   clopidrogel (Plavix)
_____ 6.   tenecteplase (TNKase)
_____ 7.   tirofiban (Aggrastat)
_____ 8.   reteplase (Retavase)
_____ 9.   epoietin alfa (Epogen, Procrit)
_____ 10.   eptifibatide (Integrilin)
_____ 11.   heparin
_____ 12.   oprelvekin (Neumega)
_____ 13.   aspirin
_____ 14.   enoxaparin (Lovenox)

A.   Thrombin inhibitor
B.   Clotting factor synthesis inhibitor
C.   Antiplatelet
D.   Thrombolytic
E.   Colony-stimulating factor

MEDICATION SAFETY PRACTICE

1.   The recommended dose of oprelvekin (Neumega) is 50 mcg/kg once daily. The correct dose of this drug for an adult who weighs 154 pounds is _____ mcg.

2.   Vitamin K is the antidote for _____.

3.   Rubbing the injection site after administering subcutaneous heparin is likely to cause _____.

4.   Colony-stimulating factors increase the patient's risk for hypertension, blood clots, strokes, and heart attacks because of increased blood _____ and _____ retention.

PRACTICE QUIZ

1. Which statement best demonstrates a patient's understanding of how warfarin (Coumadin) works to help after heart valve replacement surgery? *(Select all that apply.)*
   - _____ A. "It will thin out my blood so that it won't clot anymore."
   - _____ B. "It will make me bruise and bleed more easily, so I must be careful."
   - _____ C. "It will dissolve the clots that have formed in my heart."
   - _____ D. "New clots will not form as easily in my heart valves."
   - _____ E. "Any clots that I still have will not get any bigger."
   - _____ F. "I will feel the cold weather more because my blood is thinner now."

_____ 2. Which lab test does the nurse use to monitor the effectiveness of heparin administration to a patient who has had a venous thromboembolism (VTE)?
   - A. Prothrombin time (PT)
   - B. Activated partial prothrombin time (APPT)
   - C. Activated partial thromboplastin time (aPTT)
   - D. International normalized ratio (INR)

3. The nurse instructs a patient who is taking warfarin (Coumadin) therapy to avoid which foods? *(Select all that apply.)*
   - _____ A. Grapefruit
   - _____ B. Fava beans
   - _____ C. Spinach
   - _____ D. Bananas
   - _____ E. Kale
   - _____ F. Oranges
   - _____ G. Broccoli

_____ 4. A patient on renal dialysis who is anemic is most likely to be administered which medication?
   - A. Oprelvekin (Neumega)
   - B. Alteplase/t-PA (Activase)
   - C. Clopidogrel (Plavix)
   - D. Epoietin alfa (Epogen, Procrit)

_____ 5. A patient who is taking a clotting factor synthesis inhibitor such as warfarin (Coumadin) should be monitored for which serious adverse effect?
   - A. Decreased clotting times
   - B. Upset stomach, diarrhea, and fever
   - C. Headaches that are severe and will not go away
   - D. Increased viscosity of the blood

6. What are important lifespan considerations for an older adult who is taking warfarin (Coumadin)? *(Select all that apply.)*
   - _____ A. Aspirin increases the action of warfarin.
   - _____ B. Statin drugs decrease the action of warfarin.
   - _____ C. Older adults are more likely to develop bruises and bleeding.
   - _____ D. Sucralfate (Carafate) increases the effect of warfarin.
   - _____ E. Older adults need more frequent monitoring of the international normalized ratio (INR).

_____ 7. Which important instruction does the nurse include when teaching patients about colony-stimulating factor therapy?
   - A. Tell the patient that weight gain of more than 2 pounds a month should be reported to the prescriber.
   - B. Teach the patient how to administer intramuscular injections correctly.
   - C. Remind the patient to keep scheduled laboratory appointments for blood tests to monitor therapy.
   - D. Instruct the patient to take this medication with adequate amounts of liquid.

_____ 8. Several patients on the unit are receiving heparin. Which medication must be available on the unit to use as an antidote?
   - A. Epoietin alfa (Epogen)
   - B. Enoxaparin (Lovenox)
   - C. Vitamin K (AquaMEPHYTON)
   - D. Protamine sulfate

_____ 9.   Before administering a thrombolytic
           drug, the nurse assesses for which abso-
           lute contraindication?
           A.   Chronic peptic ulcer disease
           B.   Recent spinal or cerebral surgery
           C.   Blood pressure of 150/92 mm Hg
           D.   Current use of warfarin (Coumadin)
                or aspirin

Drugs for Asthma and Other Respiratory Problems

LEARNING ACTIVITIES

Matching

Match the correct drug category on the right with the correct medication names on the left. (Answers will be used more than once.)

_____ 1. beclomethasone (QVAR)

_____ 2. albuterol (Proventil)

_____ 3. theophylline (Theo-Dur)

_____ 4. triamcinolone (Azmacort)

_____ 5. salmeterol (Serevent)

_____ 6. fluticasone (Flovent)

_____ 7. aminophylline (Truphylline)

_____ 8. ipratropium (Atrovent)

_____ 9. budesonide (Pulmicort)

_____ 10. formoterol (Foradil)

_____ 11. terbutaline (Brethine)

_____ 12. cromolyn sodium (Intal)

_____ 13. tiotropium (Spiriva)

_____ 14. montelukast sodium (Singulair)

_____ 15. nedocromil sodium (Tilade)

_____ 16. zafirlukast (Accolate)

A. Short-acting beta$_2$ agonist
B. Long-acting beta$_2$ agonist
C. Cholinergic antagonist
D. Methylxanthine
E. Inhaled corticosteroid
F. Mast cell stabilizer
G. Leukotriene inhibitor

Terminology Review

Match the term on the right with its correct description on the left. (Answers will be used only once.)

_____ 17. Air sacs in the lungs where oxygen moves into the blood

_____ 18. Airway obstruction disease caused by constriction and inflammation

_____ 19. Sound of air moving through narrowed airways

_____ 20. Drug that reduces the thickness of mucus

_____ 21. Open center of a hollow airway

_____ 22. Inflammation of the airways

_____ 23. Disease where the elasticity of alveoli is greatly reduced

_____ 24. Tightening of pulmonary smooth muscle, resulting in narrowed airways

_____ 25. Drug that relaxes the smooth muscle around airways, causing the center openings to enlarge

A. Lumen
B. Alveoli
C. Bronchitis
D. Asthma
E. Mucolytic
F. Emphysema
G. Wheeze
H. Bronchodilator
I. Bronchoconstriction

MEDICATION SAFETY PRACTICE

1. Asthma medication that is used only during an acute episode is known as a _____ drug.

2. The most dangerous side effect of methylxanthines is cardiac and central nervous system _____.

3. The nurse must check and ensure that the patient using an oral inhaler knows the proper technique for using it, and for a _____, if one is ordered.

4. If a patient is taking more than one type of inhaled drug, the _____ drug should be given at least 5 minutes before the other drug.

PRACTICE QUIZ

_____ 1. Symptom severity in a patient with asthma or chronic bronchitis is assessed by using which method?
   A. FEV_1
   B. PERF
   C. PEEP
   D. CPAP

_____ 2. A patient who is taking a methylxanthine bronchodilator must be observed for which serious adverse effect?
   A. Nervousness
   B. Bradycardia
   C. Hypotension
   D. Seizures

_____ 3. Which important point should be included when teaching patients about the use of long-acting beta$_2$-adrenergic agonists?
   A. "Use this medication whenever you have new symptoms of wheezing."
   B. "Take an extra dose of this medication if your symptoms worsen."
   C. "Take this medication even when symptoms are not present."
   D. "Omit your daily dose of this medication if you are wheezing."

_____ 4. A child weighing 44 pounds has theophylline (Theo-Dur) prescribed every 6 hours. The recommended children's dosage range is 3-5 mg/kg every 6 hours. What is the correct dosage range for this patient?
   A. 20-40 mg
   B. 40-60 mg
   C. 60-100 mg
   D. 100-140 mg

_____ 5. What are common side effects associated with inhaled anti-inflammatory drugs? *(Select all that apply.)*
   _____ A. Bad taste
   _____ B. Mouth dryness
   _____ C. Seizures
   _____ D. Leukopenia
   _____ E. Oral infection

_____ 6. Before administering an inhaled corticosteroid, it is important for the nurse to do what?
   A. Teach the patient how to use the inhaler or spacer.
   B. Teach the patient to expect nervousness after using.
   C. Prime a new canister of nedocromil (Tilade) once before use.
   D. Administer inhaled corticosteroid agents before bronchodilators.

_____ 7. What important instruction does the nurse teach a patient who is taking guaifenesin (Mucinex)?
   A. "This medication is given to treat acetaminophen overdose."
   B. "This medication will thin your mucus and make it easier to cough up."
   C. "This medication can cause an oral infection called 'thrush'."
   D. "This medication is used with a nebulizer facemask."

Drugs for Nausea, Vomiting, Diarrhea, and Constipation

chapter

19

LEARNING ACTIVITIES

Terminology Review

Match the definitions on the right with their correct terms on the left. (Answers will be used only once.)

_____ 1. Antiemetic

_____ 2. Chemoreceptor

_____ 3. Constipation

_____ 4. Diarrhea

_____ 5. Emesis

_____ 6. Mechanoreceptors

_____ 7. Nausea

_____ 8. Peristalsis

_____ 9. Retching

_____ 10. Vestibular apparatus

_____ 11. Vomiting

A. Frequent watery bowel movements
B. Act or results of vomiting
C. Tension receptors in the bowel that initiate vomiting
D. Forcing stomach contents up through the esophagus and out of the mouth
E. Urge to vomit
F. Labored respiration with the contraction of the abdomen, chest wall, and diaphragm
G. Sensory nerve cells responding to intestinal chemical stimuli and toxins
H. Inner ear structures associated with balance and position sensing
I. Bowel movements that are infrequent and difficult or painful
J. Mass movements in the colon
K. Drugs that prevent or control nausea

Matching

Match the drug category on the right with the correct drug names on the left. (Answers will be used more than once.)

_____ 12. docusate (Colace)

_____ 13. loperamide (Imodium)

_____ 14. prochlorperazine (Compazine)

_____ 15. bismuth subsalicylate (Pepto-Bismol)

_____ 16. meclizine (Dramamine)

_____ 17. difenoxin with atropine (Motofen)

_____ 18. lactulose (Cephulac)

_____ 19. diphenoxylate with atropine (Lomotil)

_____ 20. bisacodyl (Dulcolax)

_____ 21. calcium polycarbophil (FiberCon)

_____ 22. scopolamine (L-hyoscine)

_____ 23. granisetron (Kytril)

_____ 24. metoclopramide (Reglan)

_____ 25. castor oil (Emulsoil)

A. Antidiarrheal drug
B. Antiemetic drug
C. Drug for constipation

MEDICATION SAFETY PRACTICE

1. A patient is to receive 35 mg of promethazine (Phenergan) IM. The vial that is available contains 50 mg/mL. How much promethazine will be given to the patient? _____ mL

2. List three causes of constipation.

3. List five symptoms of neuroleptic malignant syndrome.

PRACTICE QUIZ

____ 1. Which drug is likely to be the most helpful in controlling nausea and vomiting in a patient receiving chemotherapy?
A. Metoclopramide (Reglan)
B. Trimethobenzamide (Tigan)
C. Scopolamine (L-hyoscine)
D. Ondansetron (Zofran)

____ 2. Which drug for the control of nausea and vomiting is contraindicated in a patient who has a history of depression?
A. Promethazine (Phenergan)
B. Prochlorperazine (Compazine)
C. Scopolamine (L-hyoscine)
D. Metoclopramide (Reglan)

____ 3. After continued administration of promethazine (Phenergan) or prochlorperazine (Compazine), which laboratory result does the nurse monitor carefully?
A. Blood urea nitrogen (BUN)
B. Complete blood count (CBC)
C. International normalized ratio (INR)
D. Activated partial thromboplastin time (aPTT)

____ 4. An older adult woman who has problems with constipation wants to know which drug is safe for her to take on a daily or alternate-day schedule. Which drug will the nurse recommend?
A. Polyethylene glycol (MiraLax)
B. Castor oil (Emulsoil)
C. Sodium phosphate (Fleet Enema)
D. Psyllium (Metamucil)

____ 5. A patient with diabetes is advised to take a laxative every other day if no bowel movement occurs. Which laxative is contraindicated for this patient?
A. Bisacodyl (Dulcolax)
B. Lactulose (Cephulac)
C. Polyethylene glycol (MiraLax)
D. Magnesium hydroxide (Milk of Magnesia)

____ 6. An older adult who is taking an antiemetic drug requires additional monitoring for which side effects? *(Select all that apply.)*
____ A. Confusion
____ B. Shuffling gait
____ C. Diarrhea
____ D. Excessive drooling
____ E. Trembling

____ 7. Which statement indicates the patient has understood how to achieve the best response from medications for chemotherapy-induced nausea?
A. "I will take an antiemetic medication 30 minutes before meals."
B. "I will take this medication every night with a small glass of wine."
C. "I will take this medication within 1 hour after chemotherapy begins."
D. "The lip smacking and tongue movements I am experiencing are expected effects."

____ 8. After administering a medication for constipation to a patient, what is most important for the nurse to do?
A. Instruct the patient to restrict oral fluids.
B. Remind the patient to decrease his or her activity level.
C. Assess the patient for abdominal distention.
D. Assess the patient's fasting blood sugar.

9. A patient who experiences toxic megacolon after taking antimotility drugs would exhibit which signs and symptoms? *(Select all that apply.)*
____ A. Bradycardia
____ B. Fever
____ C. Abdominal pain
____ D. Distended abdomen
____ E. Hypervolemia

Drugs for Gastric Ulcers and Reflux

LEARNING ACTIVITIES

Terminology Review

Match each description on the right with its correct term on the left. (Answers will be used only once.)

_____ 1. Antacids

_____ 2. Barrett's esophagus

_____ 3. Dyspepsia

_____ 4. Lower esophageal sphincter (LES)

_____ 5. Esophagogastroduodenoscopy (EGD)

_____ 6. Gastroesophageal reflux disease (GERD)

_____ 7. Gastric ulcer

_____ 8. *Helicobacter pylori*

_____ 9. H_2 blocker

_____ 10. Peritonitis

_____ 11. Regurgitation

A. Indigestion
B. Open sore in the stomach lining
C. Upper endoscopy exam of the esophagus, stomach, and small intestine
D. Complication of severe chronic GERD
E. Esophageal irritation due to stomach acid backing up
F. Drugs that block the effects of histamine
G. Backward flow of stomach contents
H. Inflammation of the abdominal cavity
I. Bacteria that cause gastric inflammation
J. Drugs that neutralize stomach acids
K. Muscular ring located where the esophagus joins the stomach

Multiple Choice

_____ 12. What percentage of people in the U.S. develop an ulcer during their lifetime?
A. 5%
B. 10%
C. 15%
D. 20%

_____ 13. Of the following causes of gastric ulcers, which one is primary?
A. Stress
B. Diet
C. Excess gastric acid
D. *H. pylori*

_____ 14. Which weakened sphincter muscle causes gastroesophageal reflux disease (GERD)?
   A. Anal
   B. Upper esophageal
   C. Pyloric
   D. Lower esophageal

15. Which dietary factors contribute to reflux? (*Select all that apply.*)
   _____ A. Caffeine
   _____ B. Nicotine
   _____ C. Chewing gum
   _____ D. Chocolate
   _____ E. Black pepper
   _____ F. Alcohol
   _____ G. Red meats
   _____ H. Peppermint
   _____ I. Small meals
   _____ J. Leafy green vegetables
   _____ K. Eggs

MEDICATION SAFETY PRACTICE

1. Patients taking large doses of antacids containing calcium or aluminum salts over a long period of time are at risk for developing _____.

2. Patients taking milk of magnesia for indigestion over a long period of time are likely to develop _____.

3. Antacids such as Alka-Seltzer or Bromo-Seltzer are contraindicated for patients who have _____.

4. Bismuth subsalicylate (Pepto-Bismol) is contraindicated in children because of the risk for developing _____.

PRACTICE QUIZ

1. Which lab tests does the nurse monitor for patients who are taking nizatidine (Axid) or cimetidine (Tagamet)? *(Select all that apply.)*
   ____ A. Complete blood count
   ____ B. Liver function tests
   ____ C. Electrolytes
   ____ D. Urinalysis
   ____ E. Pulmonary function tests

____ 2. A 14-year-old patient who weighs 143 pounds is prescribed clarithromycin (Biaxin) for *H. pylori* infection. The recommended children's dose is 15 mg/kg orally in 2 divided doses. What is the correct dose in milligrams for *each* of the doses given in one day? _____ mg

3. Long-term use of proton pump inhibitors can lead to which conditions? *(Select all that apply.)*
   ____ A. Gastric infections
   ____ B. Bowel obstruction
   ____ C. Drowsiness
   ____ D. Anemia
   ____ E. Halitosis

____ 4. Which statement demonstrates a patient's understanding of therapy with cytoprotective drugs for treatment of gastroesophageal reflux disease (GERD)?
   A. "I will take this medicine until it relieves my symptoms."
   B. "This drug will be a life-long treatment for my stomach problems."
   C. "I need to keep my vegetable and fruit intake down while I'm on this medication."
   D. "I must take this drug for as long as my doctor prescribes it."

____ 5. During a follow-up assessment of a patient taking metoclopramide (Reglan) for treatment of GERD, the nurse observes an elevated temperature, respiratory distress, tachycardia, diaphoresis, and urinary incontinence. What is the nurse's priority action for this situation?
   A. Check the patient's medical record for drug allergies.
   B. Notify the prescriber.
   C. Give the antidote for metoclopramide.
   D. Place the patient on a cooling blanket.

____ 6. An older adult has been prescribed cimetidine (Tagamet). What is a lifespan consideration for this patient?
   A. A black tongue or bowel movement is a common effect of this medication.
   B. Due to decreased calcium absorption, hip fractures are more common.
   C. Older adults are more likely to experience dizziness and confusion.
   D. This patient should be taught how to avoid excessive exposure to the sun.

____ 7. A patient asks the nurse how the proton pump inhibitor lansoprazole (Prevacid) will help the symptoms of GERD. How does the nurse respond?
   A. "It prevents stimulation of the pumps in your stomach that produce acid."
   B. "It blocks the action of acid-secreting cells in your stomach."
   C. "It neutralizes acids in your stomach to decrease irritation."
   D. "It coats the mucosal lining of your stomach."

____ 8. Which patient statement best indicates a correct understanding of why the antibiotic clarithromycin (Biaxin) has been prescribed along with another medication for ulcers?
   A. "It treats infection with *H. pylori*."
   B. "It is effective against inflammation in the stomach."
   C. "It prevents peritonitis in the event of stomach perforation."
   D. "It treats fever associated with neuroleptic malignant syndrome."

Drugs for Seizures

LEARNING ACTIVITIES

Crossword Puzzle: Common Drug Names

Complete the puzzle by identifying the trade names of the antiseizure drugs that are described below in generic form.

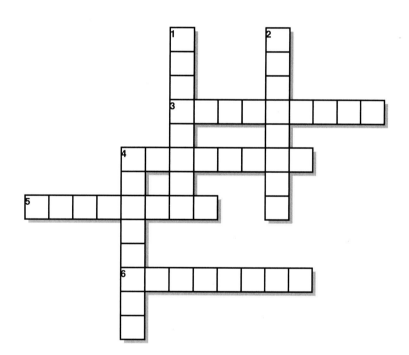

Across
3. gabapentin
4. valproic acid
5. primadone
6. carbamazepine

Down
1. clonazepam
2. ethosuximide
4. phenytoin

Terminology Review

Match the descriptions on the right with their correct terms on the left. (Answers will be used only once.)

_____ 1. Epilepsy

_____ 2. Myoclonic seizure

_____ 3. Seizure

_____ 4. Partial seizure

_____ 5. Aura

_____ 6. Status epilepticus

_____ 7. Absence seizure

_____ 8. Tonic-clonic seizure

_____ 9. Atonic seizure

_____ 10. Postictal phase

_____ 11. Generalized seizure

A. Blank stare, chewing movements, lasting less than 29 seconds

B. Sudden loss of muscle tone followed by confusion

C. Tingling, smell, or emotional changes occurring before a seizure

D. Brain disorder causing recurrent unprovoked seizures

E. Electrical discharges from both sides of the brain

F. Brief muscle jerk due to abnormal brain activity

G. Abnormal brain activity that starts in one part, may spread to the entire brain

H. Interval following a seizure featuring confusion, headache, and fatigue

I. Uncontrolled brain activity that may result in physical convulsion

J. Prolonged seizure or series of repeated seizures in a short interval

K. Stiffening or rigidity of arm and leg muscles with loss of consciousness

MEDICATION SAFETY PRACTICE

_____ 1. What can the nurse do to reduce nausea and vomiting in a patient who is taking carbamazepine (Tegretol)?
   A. Give the medication early in the morning, before breakfast.
   B. Administer the drug at bedtime.
   C. Give the medication with food.
   D. Give the drug with an antacid.

2. Which are essential aspects of care for a patient who is experiencing a tonic-clonic seizure? *(Select all that apply.)*
   _____ A. Help the person to the floor.
   _____ B. Loosen clothing around the neck.
   _____ C. Place a padded tongue blade in the mouth.
   _____ D. Turn the person to the side.
   _____ E. Remove any sharp objects.
   _____ F. Administer an immediate oral dose of antiseizure medication.

_____ 3. Which two drugs that are given to control seizures may become habit-forming?
   A. Carbamazepine (Tegretol) and valproic acid (Depakote)
   B. Phenytoin (Dilantin) and ethosuximide (Zarontin)
   C. Primidone (Mysoline) and lamotrigine (Lamictal)
   D. Phenobarbital (Luminal) and clonazepam (Klonopin)

List the medical term for each side effect of antiseizure medication below.

4. Loss of coordination, clumsiness:_____

5. Double vision: _____

6. Involuntary movements of the eyes: _____

7. Excessive growth of gum tissue:_____

8. Low platelet count: _____

9. Low white blood cell count: _____

PRACTICE QUIZ

_____ 1. Which statement demonstrates a patient's understanding of therapy with valproic acid (Depakote)?
A. "As soon as I stop having seizures, I will quit taking these pills."
B. "If I miss a dose, I need to take it as soon as possible, but not if it would be doubling a regularly scheduled dose."
C. "Since I have partial seizures, I only need to take part of one of these tablets."
D. "If I notice slowed wound healing, I will call my doctor right away."

_____ 2. A patient taking phenytoin should be instructed to call the prescriber immediately if the patient develops what condition?
A. Excessive growth of hair in areas not normally hairy
B. Overgrowth of gum tissue
C. Difficulty coordinating movements
D. Drowsiness

_____ 3. The nurse should plan to have which drug immediately available in the event a patient experiences status epilepticus?
A. Diazepam (Valium)
B. Phenytoin (Dilantin)
C. Carbamazepine (Tegretol)
D. Valproic acid (Depakote)

_____ 4. Good oral hygiene is important for patients who are taking phenytoin (Dilantin) over long periods of time because of what side effect?
A. Diplopia
B. Nystagmus
C. Hypertrichosis
D. Gingival hyperplasia

_____ 5. Which consideration is most important to remember for adolescents who are taking a first-line drug for generalized seizures?
A. They often require decreased doses because of growth changes.
B. They often require decreased doses because of hormonal changes.
C. Sometimes they stop taking the medication to avoid gum changes.
D. They often take extra doses to avoid noticeable skin changes.

_____ 6. Which instruction is most appropriate for the nurse to teach a pregnant patient who is taking a second-line drug for seizures?
A. Dizziness is more common when taking lamotrigine (Lamictal).
B. Reduce your folic acid intake when taking lamotrigine (Lamictal).
C. Primidone (Mysoline) may cause clotting problems in newborns.
D. Phenobarbital (Luminal) is associated with large-for-gestational-age fetuses.

_____ 7. The nurse is obtaining a list of home medications for a patient who will be taking phenytoin (Dilantin) and an anticoagulant. What is the possible interaction between these two drugs?
A. The effect of anticoagulants is decreased.
B. Phenytoin tends to block the effect of anticoagulants.
C. The dosage of phenytoin may need to be increased.
D. The patient is at higher risk for bleeding.

_____ 8. A patient experiences a seizure that lasts longer than 30 minutes. This situation is recognized as what kind of seizure?
A. Complex seizure
B. Status epilepticus
C. Partial seizure with secondary generalization
D. Myoclonic seizure

Drugs for Depression, Anxiety, and Psychosis

LEARNING ACTIVITIES

Crossword Puzzle: Common Drug Names

Complete the crossword puzzle by identifying the correct trade names of each drug described below in generic form.

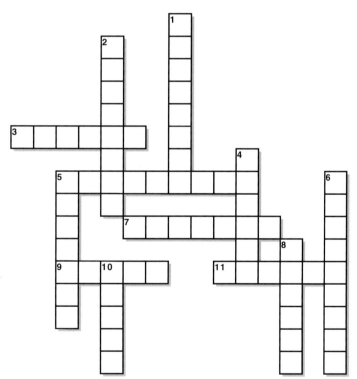

Across
3. fluoxetine
5. lithium carbonate
7. trazodone
9. paroxetine
11. thiothixene

Down
1. clonazepam
2. duloxetine
4. citalopram
5. escitalopram
6. risperidone
8. diazepam
10. alprazolam

Terminology Review

Match the descriptions on the right with their correct terms on the left. (Answers will be used only once.)

_____ 1. Anxiety

_____ 2. Bipolar disorder

_____ 3. Depression

_____ 4. Delusions

_____ 5. Dysthymia

_____ 6. Hallucinations

_____ 7. Illusions

_____ 8. Major depression

_____ 9. Mania

_____ 10. Obsessive-compulsive disorder

_____ 11. Panic disorder

_____ 12. Post-traumatic stress disorder

_____ 13. Psychosis

A. Alternating episodes of mania and depression
B. Fixed false beliefs of opinions that are resistant to reason
C. Feeling of dread about a perceived danger or threat
D. Incorrect mental representations of misinterpreted events
E. Feelings of sadness, despair, loss of energy, and difficulty coping
F. Sensory perceptions not actually present
G. Obsessive thoughts and compulsive actions
H. Distorted thinking, hallucinations, and reduced ability to feel normal emotions
I. Persistently low moods; less severe than depression
J. Unexpected attacks of anxiety or terror lasting 15-30 minutes
K. Extremely elevated mood with mental and physical hyperactivity
L. Anxiety disorder caused by serious traumatic events
M. Persistent low mood and lack of pleasure in life with an increased risk of suicide

MEDICATION SAFETY PRACTICE

1. Patients taking venlafaxine, duloxetine, or bupropion are at risk for

    _____ .

2. Patients on mirtazapine are at increased risk for infection because of

    _____ .

3. Because of their abuse potential, _____ drugs are contraindicated for patients with a substance abuse disorder.

4. Patients taking quetiapine may experience an alteration in

    _____ .

5. A patient has been prescribed chlorpromazine (Thorazine) 35 mg IM STAT. The medication is available in vials of 50 mg/2 mL. How many mL should be administered to the patient? _____ mL

PRACTICE QUIZ

____ 1. A patient who has been taking the benzo-diazepine chlordiazepoxide (Librium) for anxiety reports after 2 weeks of therapy that she is feeling much calmer. This is a result of the enhanced inhibitory effects of which neurotransmitter?
A. Serotonin
B. Gamma-aminobutyric acid
C. Dopamine
D. Norepinephrine

____ 2. A patient who was prescribed lorazepam (Ativan) for 2 months suddenly stopped taking it because she "felt so much better." Now she reports restlessness, weakness, and insomnia. The nurse will instruct her to call the prescriber and make an appointment immediately because of what risk associated with benzodiazepine withdrawal?
A. Sedation
B. Hypotension
C. Seizures
D. Stevens-Johnson syndrome

____ 3. A patient who is in her second trimester of pregnancy is experiencing emotional difficulty at home and asks her physician for a prescription for lorazepam (Ativan) to help her cope. Why is this drug contraindicated for this patient?
A. It can cause birth defects.
B. The fetus can become dependent on the drug.
C. The risk of pre-eclampsia is increased.
D. It might make the patient miscarry.

____ 4. A patient who has been taking sertraline (Zoloft) daily for 10 days reports that the medication has not helped with anxiety. What does the nurse tell the patient?
A. "This is a low dose and the prescriber will be contacted to request an increase."
B. "You should probably be taking a benzodiazepine for your condition."
C. "Another medication should be added to your regimen in order to get good results."
D. "You must give the drug more time because it is usually takes several weeks to be effective."

____ 5. A patient has begun treatment with 25 mg of chlorpromazine (Thorazine) BID. The nurse instructs the patient to be sure to practice which precaution?
A. Do not take the medication with grapefruit juice.
B. Record daily weights to monitor for retained fluid.
C. Change positions and get up slowly.
D. Check fasting blood sugar daily.

____ 6. A patient has recently begun taking citalopram (Celexa) for symptoms of depression. The nurse will monitor the patient for which common side effects? *(Select all that apply.)*
____ A. Insomnia
____ B. Anorexia
____ C. Dry mouth
____ D. Facial grimacing
____ E. Increased sweating

____ 7. A group of individuals is participating in a support session to help with depression. Which patient statement would warrant an immediate notification of his or her health care provider?
A. "I still have feelings of extreme sadness every single day."
B. "When will this medication start to work? I still cry a lot."
C. "My mouth is so dry, I wish I never started taking my medication."
D. "If things don't improve, I'll have no reason to live anymore."

____ 8. A patient who has taken chlorpromazine (Thorazine) has developed symptoms of muscle rigidity, elevated temperature, increased respiratory rate, and elevated pulse and blood pressure. In addition, the patient has become less responsive to verbal stimuli. Which adverse reaction has this patient developed?
A. Tardive dyskinesia
B. Neutropenia
C. Neuroleptic malignant syndrome
D. Myocarditis

_____ 9.   Before giving clozapine (Clozaril) to a patient, the nurse assesses the patient's smoking history. What is the reason for this assessment?
A.   Hand tremors may cause self-injury while smoking.
B.   Smoking increases the risk of tardive dyskinesia.
C.   Smoking may decrease the effectiveness of clozapine.
D.   Smoking increases the risk of dementia.

_____ 10. Which statement made by a patient best indicates that the patient correctly understands the correct use of olanzapine (Zyprexa)?
A.   "I won't worry if this drug causes my urine to turn pinkish brown."
B.   "I won't take this drug with grapefruit juice to avoid excessive blood levels."
C.   "I can drink a glass of wine at night to help me relax and sleep better."
D.   "Suntanning is acceptable, as long as I do not use a tanning bed."

_____ 11. An older adult has been taking lithium and develops nausea and vomiting. Which nursing intervention is most appropriate?
A.   Contact the prescriber for possible parenteral fluids.
B.   Remind the patient to restrict fluid intake.
C.   Hold the lithium until the nausea subsides.
D.   Instruct the patient about ways to restrict sodium intake.

Drugs for Alzheimer's and Parkinson's Disease

chapter

23

LEARNING ACTIVITIES

Matching

Match each generic drug name on the right with its correct trade name on the left. (Answers will be used only once.)

____ 1. Namenda

____ 2. Aricept

____ 3. Excelon

____ 4. Reminyl

A. galantamine
B. rivastigmine
C. memantine
D. donepezil

Match each category of drug on the right with the correct drug on the left. (Categories will be used more than once.)

____ 5. entacapone (Comtan)

____ 6. selegiline (Eldepryl)

____ 7. pramipexole (Mirapex)

____ 8. apomorphine (Apokyn)

____ 9. tolcapone (Tasmar)

____ 10. rasagiline (Azilect)

____ 11. benztropine (Cogentin)

____ 12. ropinirole (Requip)

____ 13. trihexyphenidyl (Artane)

____ 14. bromocriptine (Parlodel)

____ 15. carbidopa/levodopa (Sinemet)

A. Dopamine antagonist
B. COMT inhibitor
C. MAO-B inhibitor
D. Anticholinergic

MEDICATION SAFETY PRACTICE

____ 1. Before administering apomorphine (Apikinin), the nurse obtains appropriate equipment in order to administer the medication by which route?
   A. Oral
   B. Intravenous
   C. Intramuscular
   D. Subcutaneous

_____ 2. Due to the progressive effects of Alzheimer's disease, what must the nurse assess in a patient with the disease before administering oral medication?
A. Intake and output for the day
B. Vital signs
C. Ability to swallow
D. Daily weight

_____ 3. What must family and patients be taught about administration of timed-release forms of medication?
A. Always give with food.
B. Do not give with grapefruit juice.
C. Do not open or crush.
D. Take with at least one full glass of water.

4. A patient with Parkinson's disease is prescribed ropinirole (Requip) 0.5 mg PO. The drug is available in scored tablets of 0.25 mg. How many tablets are given to the patient? _____ tablet(s)

PRACTICE QUIZ

____ 1. Which drug for Alzheimer's disease reduces the activity of the enzyme acetylcholinesterase that breaks down acetylcholine in the synapses of neurons?
A. Memantine (Namenda)
B. Galantamine (Reminyl)
C. Entacapone (Comtan)
D. Selegiline (Eldepryl)

2. A patient who is taking donepezil (Aricept) For Alzheimer's disease should be monitored for symptoms of which adverse effects? *(Select all that apply.)*
____ A. Seizures
____ B. Tachycardia
____ C. Atrial fibrillation
____ D. Muscle weakness
____ E. Weight gain

____ 3. A nursing assistant in a long-term care facility reports that a patient with Alzheimer's disease choked several times during breakfast this morning. Which action is best to take before giving sustained-release galantamine (Razadyne) to this patient?
A. Crush the medication and place it in applesauce or softened ice cream.
B. Determine which food the patient enjoys and open the capsule onto it.
C. Assess the patient's swallowing ability before giving the medication.
D. Obtain the patient's height and weight to determine caloric needs.

____ 4. Which statement by a family member indicates a correct understanding about the use of memantine (Namenda) for Alzheimer's disease?
A. "I will administer this medication on an empty stomach."
B. "This medication is also available in a skin patch."
C. "This should improve the ability to perform complex tasks."
D. "I will keep the medication stored in a safe location."

____ 5. An older woman with Alzheimer's disease is very frail, weighing only 94 pounds. The nurse is reviewing the patient's medication record and notes that donepezil (Aricept) 10 mg PO at bedtime has been prescribed. What is the best action for the nurse to take?
A. Administer the medication with food to avoid GI upset.
B. Change the administration time to every morning.
C. Ask the patient which food she would like the medication with.
D. Consult with the prescriber about the drug dosage.

6. A patient is ordered pramipexole (Mirapex) to be given in three divided doses for a daily total of 4.5 mg. How many mg will each individual dose be?
_____ mg

____ 7. A patient who is taking entacapone (Comtan) reports feeling weak and achy recently. What question does the nurse ask the patient next?
A. "What color is your urine?"
B. "Have you lost more than 5 pounds in the last month?"
C. "Do you have a fever?"
D. "What color are the whites of your eyes?"
E. "Have you had a bowel movement today?"

____ 8. A patient who is taking ropinirole (Requip) to treat Parkinson's disease should be watched carefully for which potentially dangerous effect?
A. Episodes of falling asleep suddenly
B. Malignant melanoma
C. Dyskinesia
D. Rhinorrhea

____ 9. A patient who is taking selegiline (Eldepryl) proudly announces he will be attending a college graduation party for his grandson. Which item must the patient avoid while taking this medication?
A. Beer
B. White wine
C. Potato chips
D. Pretzels

____ 10. An older adult who is taking medication for Parkinson's disease should be cautioned to use extra care when walking because of which drug response?
A. An increased risk for bradykinesia
B. Rapid increase in blood pressure
C. Confusion and hallucinations
D. Rhinorrhea and excessive drooling

Drugs for Endocrine Problems

LEARNING ACTIVITIES

Crossword Puzzle: Terminology Review

Complete the puzzle by identifying the correct words described in the clues below.

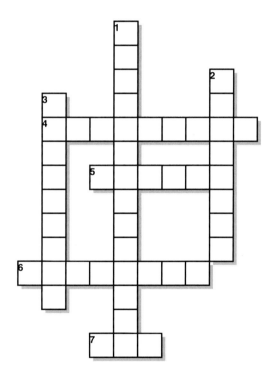

Across
4. Gland secreting hormone carried by blood
5. Enlarged thyroid gland
6. Main female sex hormone
7. Pituitary hormone; causes estrogen secretion by ovary

Down
1. Another name for hyperthyroidism
2. Beginning of menstrual cycles
3. Cessation of menstruation and ovulation

Matching

Match each perimenopausal symptom on the left with its correct cause on the right. (Causes will be used more than once.)

_____ 1. Decreased mental concentration

_____ 2. Reduced cervical mucus

_____ 3. Night sweats

_____ 4. Sleep difficulties

_____ 5. Atrophy of vaginal tissue

_____ 6. Hot flashes

_____ 7. Painful intercourse

_____ 8. Dry skin

_____ 9. Increased rate of osteoporosis

A. Reduced estrogen
B. High follicle-stimulating hormone (FSH) levels

MEDICATION SAFETY PRACTICE

1. The nurse teaches a patient about the interaction between thyroid hormone replacement drugs and warfarin (Coumadin) because of the increased risk of _____.

2. Thyroid hormone replacement drugs should never be substituted for one another due to their variation in strengths as well as the patient's _____.

3. Taking perimenopausal hormone replacement therapy (HRT) more often than prescribed, or not following instructions for timing, will increase the risk for excessive _____.

4. A child who weighs 22 pounds is prescribed levothyroxine (Levothroid) 10 mcg/kg daily. How many mcg will the child receive each day? _____ mcg

PRACTICE QUIZ

____ 1. Which statement by a patient who is taking thyroid replacement medication demonstrates a correct understanding of the therapy?
A. "As soon as my levels get back to normal, I can quit taking these pills."
B. "These pills will only serve to make me gain weight."
C. "I hope to feel better in general, and be more energetic during the day."
D. "I'll take this in the evening when I take my fiber supplement; that way I won't forget."

2. What cardiac events may result from increased activity brought about by thyroid hormone replacement (HRT)? *(Select all that apply.)*
____ A. Tamponade
____ B. Infarction
____ C. Heart block
____ D. Angina
____ E. Aortic stenosis
____ F. Heart failure

____ 3. A patient who has Graves' disease has an endocrine disorder characterized by what action?
A. The thyroid gland does not produce enough hormone.
B. The body makes antibodies to thyroid-stimulating hormone which bind to receptors.
C. Antigens produced in the blood block hormone function.
D. Slowed body metabolism causes decreased production of thyroid hormone.

____ 4. Which statement best describes the mechanism of action of thyroid-suppressing drugs?
A. Cells in the thyroid gland are killed by toxins and rendered unable to produce hormone.
B. Thiamine is destroyed and cannot connect with iodine to make hormone.
C. Hormones already formed and stored in the gland are depleted.
D. The drug combines with the enzyme responsible for connecting iodide with tyrosine.

____ 5. Before administering thyroid replacement hormones, which action is crucial?
A. Administering the medication on the same schedule as at home
B. Encouraging the patient to ask the pharmacist for a less-expensive brand
C. Administering the medication with food to decrease stomach upset
D. Dividing the prescribed medication into several doses throughout the day

____ 6. An infant has been diagnosed with congenital absence of the thyroid gland. What should the nurse emphasize during parent counseling?
A. Most thyroid medications are prepared from nonallergenic animals.
B. This medication is prescribed to promote mental and physical development.
C. This medication will need to be taken only through adolescence.
D. This medication eliminates the need for future monitoring of thyroid levels.

7. A patient is considering her options regarding use of hormone replacement therapy (HRT). The nurse teaches the patient about the possible adverse effects of HRT which include an increased risk for which conditions? *(Select all that apply.)*
____ A. Deep vein thrombosis
____ B. Myocardial infarction
____ C. Renal dysfunction
____ D. Osteoporosis and fractures
____ E. Ovarian and uterine cancers

____ 8. Which patient statement best reflects a correct understanding of hormone replacement therapy for menopausal symptoms?
A. "This drug could cause bone marrow suppression."
B. "If I develop leg swelling, I should contact my prescriber."
C. "Smoking will decrease the effectiveness of the hormone."
D. "Now I will no longer need my annual mammograms."

Drugs for Diabetes

LEARNING ACTIVITIES

Crossword Puzzle: Terminology Review

Complete the puzzle by identifying the correct terms described in the clues below.

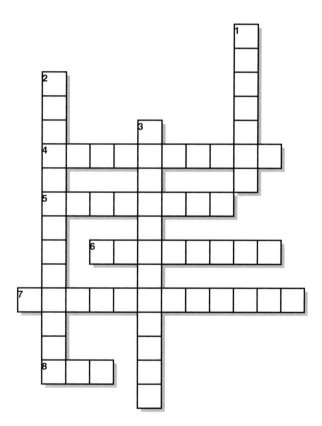

Across
4. Normal range of fasting blood glucose
5. Hormone secreted by pancreas alpha cells
6. Type of diabetes related to reduced insulin effectiveness
7. Excessive byproduct of fat metabolism
8. Body's main chemical energy substance

Down
1. Hormone secreted by pancreas beta cells
2. Higher-than-normal blood glucose level
3. Lower-than-normal blood glucose level

Matching

Match each type of oral antidiabetic drug on the right with its correct drug name on the left. (Drug types will be used more than once.)

____ 1. pioglitazone (Actos)

____ 2. glipizide (Glucotrol)

____ 3. repaglinide (Prandin)

____ 4. glyburide (DiaBeta, Micronase)

____ 5. acarbose (Precose)

____ 6. glimepride (Amaryl)

____ 7. nateglinide (Starlix)

____ 8. glyburide, micronized (Glynase)

____ 9. metformin (Glucophage)

____ 10. miglitol (Glyset)

____ 11. rosiglitazone (Avandia)

A. Sulfonylurea
B. Meglitinide
C. Biguanide
D. Alpha-glucosidase inhibitor
E. Thiazolidinedione

MEDICATION SAFETY PRACTICE

1. The nurse will instruct the patient to rotate injection sites for insulin to minimize the risk of developing _____.

2. True or False: After inserting the needle for an insulin injection, aspiration should be done before depressing the plunger.

3. True or False: Before withdrawing insulin from the bottle or using a prefilled device, the container should be shaken vigorously to make sure the suspension is evenly distributed.

4. True or False: Prefilled pens and cartridges of insulin detemir (Levemir) should be stored at room temperature.

5. List three challenges to maintaining good control over blood glucose levels in pediatric patients.

    a. _____

    b. _____

    c. _____

PRACTICE QUIZ

____ 1. What effect are the last two trimesters of pregnancy likely to have on the insulin needs of a patient with diabetes?
A. Increase during morning hours
B. Decrease at bedtime
C. Plateau at lunchtime
D. Overall increase

2. Which conditions can result from poorly controlled diabetes? *(Select all that apply.)*
____ A. Increased risk for infection
____ B. Increased sensitivity to touch
____ C. Elevated cholesterol levels
____ D. Kidney failure
____ E. Orthostatic hypotension

____ 3. A patient with diabetes who takes gluco-phage (Metformin) has postoperative or-ders to "resume all pre-op medications." What is the priority action for the nurse?
A. Follow the orders and resume all pre-operative medications.
B. Hold all preoperative medications until verified with the pharmacy.
C. Contact the prescriber to obtain an order to hold the glucophage for 48 hours.
D. Resume only oral preoperative medications.
E. Hold oral preoperative medications until the patient has a bowel movement.

____ 4. A 68-year-old patient who is taking pio-glitazone (Actose) will have which labo-ratory test done for follow-up?
A. Pulmonary function test (PFT)
B. Alanine transaminase (ALT)
C. Thyroid-stimulating hormone (TSH)
D. Complete blood count (CBC)

____ 5. A patient has been prescribed exenatide (Byetta). Which patient statement indi-cates a correct understanding of the use of this drug?
A. "I should keep this medication in the refrigerator, not the freezer."
B. "Even if I miss breakfast, I should still take my exenatide."
C. "This medication can cause weight gain, so I'll need to eat less."
D. "This medication can cause me to feel hungrier between meals."

____ 6. At 10 AM, a patient who was given an injection of Humulin R at 7:30 AM is anxious, has cool clammy skin, and no-ticeable hand tremors. What is the most likely explanation for these symptoms?
A. The insulin is nearing the end of its duration of action.
B. The insulin is having its peak effect, causing hypoglycemia.
C. The patient likely ingested an exces-sive amount of carbohydrates.
D. The patient has received an insuffi-cient amount of insulin.

____ 7. Which is the best action to ensure proper dosing before administering 50 units of Humulin N?
A. Use a 5-mL syringe and administer 0.5 mL.
B. Administer 50 units of insulin glargine.
C. Ensure the vial contents are complete-ly clear.
D. Use a 50-unit or a 100-unit syringe.

____ 8. Which approach to patient teaching is most likely to be effective for a newly di-agnosed patient with type 1 diabetes?
A. Plan to provide one extended teach-ing session for the patient.
B. Provide a variety of insulin syringes for the patient to examine.
C. Ask the patient and the patient's care-giver to demonstrate back to you.
D. Remind the patient that amputation could result if appropriate doses are not given.

____ 9. A nurse is observing a colleague prepare to administer insulin by the subcutaneous route. The nurse intervenes and provides additional instruction under which cir-cumstance?
A. The colleague selects a 1-inch, 22-gauge needle for the injection.
B. The colleague inserts the needle at a 45-degree angle for a thin patient.
C. The colleague injects the insulin with-out first checking for a blood return.
D. The colleague withdraws the needle rapidly after the injection is complet-ed.

_____ 10. What is the correct order of steps for combining two types of insulin into one syringe? (The dose to be given is 32 units of NPH and 8 units of regular insulin.)
1. Draw up 8 units of air and inject into the regular vial.
2. Ensure there is a total of 40 units in the syringe.
3. Clean the tops of each vial with separate alcohol swabs.
4. Draw up 32 units of NPH insulin into the syringe.
5. Draw up 8 units of regular insulin into the syringe.
6. Draw up 32 units of air and inject it into the NPH vial.
A. 2, 3, 6, 1, 4, 5
B. 3, 6, 1, 5, 4, 2
C. 3, 1, 5, 6, 2, 4
D. 2, 3, 4, 1, 5, 6

_____ 11. A patient is prescribed rosiglitazone (Avandia). The nurse should monitor for which adverse effect associated specifically with this drug?
A. Lactic acidosis
B. Difficulty digesting fatty meals
C. Heart failure
D. Kidney failure

_____ 12. The nurse has been instructing a patient about oral diabetic medications. Which patient statement indicates a need for additional teaching?
A. "I will avoid drinking alcohol because I might not recognize hypoglycemia."
B. "I will need to stay out of the sun while I am taking glipizide (Glucotrol)."
C. "While I'm taking metformin (Glucophage), I can avoid the formation of lactic acid by drinking plenty of water."
D. "I will take nateglinide (Starlix) twice daily with breakfast and dinner only."

Drugs for Glaucoma

LEARNING ACTIVITIES

Terminology Review

Match the descriptions on the right with the correct terms on the left. (Answers will be used only once.)

_____ 1. Anterior chamber

_____ 2. Anterior segment

_____ 3. Aqueous humor

_____ 4. Conjunctiva

_____ 5. Glaucoma

_____ 6. Miosis

_____ 7. Mydriasis

_____ 8. Posterior chamber

_____ 9. Punctum

_____ 10. Posterior segment

_____ 11. Photoreceptors

_____ 12. Retina

_____ 13. Sclera

A. White outer layer of the eye
B. Clear membrane covering the front of the eye
C. Dilation of the pupil
D. Drains tears into the nasolacrimal sac
E. Back of the eye from the lens to the optic nerve
F. Increased intraocular pressure
G. Light-activated nerve endings
H. Clear fluid maintaining pressure and shape of the eye
I. Lining of the eye containing photoreceptors
J. Segment of the eye from the iris to the cornea
K. Constriction of the pupil
L. Part of the eye between the lens and the iris
M. Part of the eye between the lens and the cornea; contains chambers

Matching: Common Drug Names

Match the class of glaucoma drug on the right with the correct names on the left. (Types will be used more than once.)

_____ 14. apraclonidine (Iopidine)

_____ 15. carbachol (Carboptic)

_____ 16. betaxolol (Betoptic)

_____ 17. bimatoprost (Lumigan)

_____ 18. acetazolamide (Diamox)

_____ 19. levobunolol (Betagan)

_____ 20. pilocarpine (Ocusert)

_____ 21. latanoprost (Xalatan)

_____ 22. methazolamide (Neptazane)

_____ 23. carteolol (Ocupress)

_____ 24. brimonidine (Alphagan P)

_____ 25. travoprost (Travatan)

_____ 26. timolol (Timoptic)

_____ 27. dorzolamide (Trusopt)

_____ 28. echothiophate (Phospholine Iodide)

_____ 29. dipivefrin (Propine)

_____ 30. brinzolamide (Azopt)

A. Prostaglandin agonist
B. Beta blocker
C. Adrenergic agonist
D. Cholinergic
E. Carbonic anhydrase inhibitor

MEDICATION SAFETY PRACTICE

_____ 1. Why is aseptic technique used to instill eye drops?
A. The eye is sterile.
B. Eye medications are sterile.
C. The eye is not well-protected by the immune system.
D. Drug interactions may occur when multiple medications are administered.

_____ 2. Some drugs for the eye are also available as regular topical ointments. How are these formulations different?
A. Neither preparation is sterile.
B. The concentration of topical ointments is less.
C. Topical ointments are suspended in non-water–soluble carriers.
D. The particles contained in the topical ointments are larger and should not be put in the eye.

3. The action performed to reduce systemic absorption of eye medication is known as _____.

4. Prostaglandin agonists should only be used if the eye is
    _____.

5. Long-term use of beta blockers can increase the risk for
    _____.

6. In patients who have asthma or heart failure, _____
    drugs should be used with caution.

7. Patients who have taken MAO inhibitors within the last 2 weeks should not
    use _____ eye medications.

8. If a patient is to be administered another eye medication after a carbonic
    anhydrase inhibitor, there should be an interval of _____
    between instilling the two drugs.

PRACTICE QUIZ

____ 1.   When an eye appears "bloodshot," the vessels that are visible are in what part of the eye?
A. Sclera
B. Pupil
C. Aqueous humor
D. Conjunctiva

____ 2.   An older adult patient with diabetes who is taking beta blockers for glaucoma must be instructed to perform what assessment?
A. Daily weight
B. Intake and output
C. Blood glucose level
D. Urine ketones

____ 3.   Which is most important for the nurse to assess before administering a prostaglandin agent to a patient?
A. Corneal color changes
B. Excessive eyelash growth
C. Presence of cataracts
D. Whether the eye surface is intact

____ 4.   What teaching point must be included for a patient who is taking cholinergic drugs for treatment of glaucoma?
A. Wear sunglasses when reading fine print indoors.
B. Limit your fluid intake to less than 2000 mL per day.
C. Apply punctal pressure for 10 minutes to avoid systemic effects.
D. Use caution in dim lighting to prevent falls and injury.

____ 5.   A patient had an allergic reaction to a sulfa antibiotic 1 year ago. This indicates that the patient may have sensitivities to which eye medication?
A. Carbonic anhydrase inhibitors
B. Cholinergics
C. Prostaglandin agonists
D. Adrenergic blockers

____ 6.   The rationale for pressing on the inner canthus after instilling eye drops is to avoid what event?
A. Overdosage
B. Contamination
C. Systemic side effects
D. Increased intraocular pressure

____ 7.   A middle-aged patient with glaucoma is not following the prescribed regimen for instilling eye drops. He says he can see just fine and his eyes do not hurt. What factors regarding glaucoma must the nurse review with him?
A. Vision damage from glaucoma occurs painlessly.
B. When the pain from glaucoma returns, resume eye drop use.
C. When difficulty seeing occurs, resume eye drop use.
D. Your central vision would be affected first with glaucoma.

Drugs for Cancer Therapy

LEARNING ACTIVITIES

Terminology Review

Match the definitions on the right with their correct terms on the left. (Answers will be used only once.)

_____ 1. Apoptosis

_____ 2. Benign

_____ 3. Carcinogen

_____ 4. Cyclins

_____ 5. Emetogenic

_____ 6. Extravasation

_____ 7. Hyperplasia

_____ 8. Hypertrophy

_____ 9. Metastasis

_____ 10. Mitosis

_____ 11. Mucositis

_____ 12. Cytotoxic

_____ 13. Neutropenia

_____ 14. Primary tumor

_____ 15. Thrombocytopenia

_____ 16. Vesicant

A. Reduced number of platelets
B. Spread of cancer cells to other body areas
C. Tissue growth caused by an increased number of cells
D. Severe white blood cell suppression
E. Tissue growth by cell division
F. Tumor type that is usually harmless
G. Inflammation and ulcers in mucous membranes
H. Substance or event that can cause cancer development
I. Chemicals or drugs that damage tissue on direct contact
J. Tissue growth caused by increased cell size
K. Programmed cell death
L. Proteins promoting cells to divide
M. Substance that induces vomiting
N. Leakage of irritating drug into surrounding tissues
O. Cell-damaging and cell-killing effects
P. Original site where normal cells become cancer

Matching

Match the mechanism of action on the right with its correct chemotherapy drug category on the left. (Answers will be used only once.)

_____ 17. Antimetabolites

_____ 18. Antitumor antibiotics

_____ 19. Antimitotics

_____ 20. Alkylating agents

_____ 21. Topoisomerase inhibitors

A. Interfere with tubule formation
B. Cause DNA breakage and cell death
C. Fool cancer cells into using the wrong substance in cellular reactions
D. Bind DNA strands by cross-linking
E. Interrupt synthesis of DNA or RNA

Multiple Choice

22. Which drugs might be administered before chemotherapy as premedications? *(Select all that apply.)*
    _____ A. Prochlorperazine (Compazine)
    _____ B. Dexamethasone (Decadron)
    _____ C. Lorazepam (Ativan)
    _____ D. Nicotinic acid (Niacin)
    _____ E. Cephalexin (Keflex)
    _____ F. Metformin (Glucophage)

MEDICATION SAFETY PRACTICE

1. Due to the risk of absorption of chemotherapy drugs, what precautions must the nurse take in their preparation and administration? *(Select all that apply.)*
    _____ A. Eye protection
    _____ B. Mask
    _____ C. Foot covering
    _____ D. Hair covering
    _____ E. Double gloves
    _____ F. Laminar flow hood
    _____ G. Gown
    _____ H. Prophylactic interferon injections

_____ 2. In the event of an adverse or anaphylactic reaction during the administration of chemotherapy drugs, what is the nurse's priority action?
    A. Notify the primary care provider.
    B. Administer diphenhydramine (Benadryl).
    C. Prevent any more drug from entering the patient.
    D. Slow the infusion to a "keep open" rate.
    E. Discontinue the IV and apply warm packs.

3. What teaching interventions are required for a patient who has thrombocytopenia? *(Select all that apply.)*
    _____ A. Drink at least 2 liters of fluid daily.
    _____ B. Avoid dairy products.
    _____ C. Use a soft-bristle toothbrush.
    _____ D. Avoid straining with bowel movements.
    _____ E. Use enemas or suppositories to prevent constipation.
    _____ F. Maintain a daily aspirin regimen.
    _____ G. Consult the oncologist before scheduling any dental work.

PRACTICE QUIZ

_____ 1. Which regimen of antiemetics is most likely to control chemotherapy-induced nausea and vomiting?
   A. Start with prochlorperazine (Compazine) and move to more potent drugs such as ondansetron (Zofrin) or granisetron (Kytril) as needed.
   B. Administer medications on a PRN basis, not exceeding the maximum recommended dosage.
   C. Premedicate before chemotherapy administration and continue the medication on a scheduled basis.
   D. Alternate oral and parenteral routes of administration to maximize drug absorption.

_____ 2. A patient who is receiving chemotherapy is fatigued and has an oxygen saturation of 86%. The patient's red blood cell count is 1.8 million/mm³. After starting supplemental oxygen, what treatment is the prescriber most likely to order?
   A. Plasmapheresis
   B. Bone marrow transplant
   C. Platelet cell transfusion
   D. Biologic response modifier

3. Which of the following are known carcinogens? (_Select all that apply._)
   _____ A. Asbestos
   _____ B. Marijuana
   _____ C. Radiation
   _____ D. Mineral oils
   _____ E. Alcoholic beverages

_____ 4. A patient has had a mastectomy for breast cancer and will follow up with radiation treatments and chemotherapy. This is characteristic of what type of therapy?
   A. Targeted
   B. Biological response modification
   C. Hormonal manipulation
   D. Adjuvant

_____ 5. A patient who has had treatment for breast cancer should be monitored for the spread of cancer to which area?
   A. Gastrointestinal tract
   B. Lungs
   C. Pancreas
   D. Pelvis

_____ 6. A patient with cancer wants to postpone several appointments for chemotherapy. The nurse discourages postponement because the basis for scheduling chemotherapy doses is dependent on which factor?
   A. Available transportation for the patient
   B. Doctor's schedule
   C. Availability of medication from the manufacturer
   D. Maximization of cancer cells killed

_____ 7. Before administering a dose of chemotherapy, the patient's white blood cell count is checked. The results show 1.6 segmented neutrophils and 0.4 band neutrophils. What is the patient's absolute neutrophil count?
   A. 246 cells/mm³
   B. 750 cells/mm³
   C. 1270 cells/mm³
   D. 1500 cells/mm³
   E. 2000 cells/mm³

_____ 8. In an oncology clinic, several patients' pathology reports are being reviewed by the health care team. Which descriptions are most likely to apply to cancer cells?
   A. Nondifferentiated function
   B. Tight adherence
   C. Nonmigration
   D. Well-regulated growth

_____ 9. A patient is receiving chemotherapy through a peripheral IV site. Which action will most likely prevent extravasation?
   A. Apply cool compresses over the IV site during infusion.
   B. Assess the IV infusion site at least every 30 minutes.
   C. Discontinue the infusion if a brisk blood return is present.
   D. Ensure that only an advanced-practice registered nurse gives the medication.

____ 10. A patient who has undergone chemotherapy has received instruction about how to avoid infections if neutropenia develops. Which patient statement indicates a need for further teaching?
A. "I will ask someone else in my household to clean the cat litter box."
B. "I should not dig in my garden or work with house plants."
C. "I will need to avoid eating raw, fresh fruits and vegetables."
D. "I will need a platelet transfusion if my counts remain low."

____ 11. Which is essential to include when teaching patients about thrombocytopenia?
A. Playing football is acceptable if the patient wears a helmet and padding.
B. A white blood cell transfusion may be necessary if the counts remain low.
C. Do not have dental work performed without consulting your oncologist.
D. Use enemas or rectal suppositories to relieve occasional constipation.

____ 12. A woman who is 8 weeks pregnant has been informed that she has leukemia and will need to undergo chemotherapy. Which should be considered in this patient's care?
A. The patient should be encouraged to terminate her pregnancy.
B. The decision of using chemotherapy should be made by the patient.
C. Breastfeeding while taking chemotherapy is considered to be safe.
D. Chemotherapy is safer during the first trimester, while the embryo is small.

____ 13. Hormone manipulation therapy is most frequently prescribed for patients who have which type of cancer?
A. Prostate
B. Liver
C. Lung
D. Bone

____ 14. A patient with melanoma will be receiving interferon therapy. What is the expected benefit from this drug?
A. It helps cancer cells appear abnormal.
B. It increases the expression of oncogenes.
C. It increases cell division within tumors.
D. It stimulates growth of natural killer cells.

____ 15. Targeted therapies combine which aspects of treatment?
A. Gene therapy and immunotherapy
B. Cell growth inhibition and carcinogen suppression
C. Antimetabolites and antimitotic effects
D. Alkylating activity and antitumor antibody production